Out of the Lyme Light and Into the Sunlight

Birding as Therapy for the Chronically Ill

ROBERT C. BELL

Copyright © 2022 Robert C. Bell

Cataloguing data available from Library and Archives Canada
978-0-88839-747-8 [paperback]
978-0-88839-749-2 [hardcover]
978-0-88839-750-8 [epub]

Illustrations and photographs are copyrighted by the artist or the Publisher unless stated otherwise.

Printed in China

FRONT COVER ARTWORK: CANDACE OSBORNE BELL [CANDACEOBELL.COM]

PRODUCTION & DESIGN: J. Rade & M. Lamont

EDITOR: D. MARTENS

We acknowledge the support of the Government of Canada through the Canada Book Fund and the Canada Council for the Arts, and of the Province of British Columbia through the British Columbia Arts Council and the Book Publishing Tax Credit.

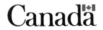 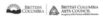

Hancock House gratefully acknowledges the Halkomelem Speaking Peoples whose unceded, shared and asserted traditional territories our offices reside upon.

Published simultaneously in Canada and the United States by
HANCOCK HOUSE PUBLISHERS LTD.
19313 Zero Avenue, Surrey, B.C. Canada V3Z 9R9
#104-4550 Birch Bay-Lynden Rd, Blaine, WA, U.S.A. 98230-9436
(800) 938-1114   Fax (800) 983-2262
www.hancockhouse.com   info@hancockhouse.com

Out of the Lyme Light and Into the Sunlight

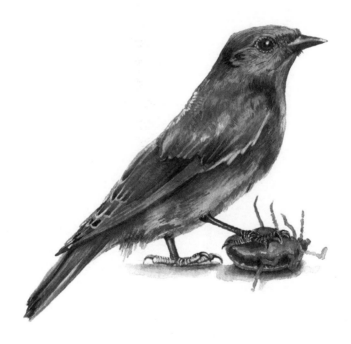

Birding as Therapy for the Chronically Ill

ROBERT C. BELL

Bob Bell's *Out of the Lyme Light and Into the Sunlight* offers the reader a wonderfully engrossing story of personal transformation in the wake of a life upended by a debilitating and enigmatic illness. Although there is no miracle cure for Lyme disease, Bell finds a way to live meaningfully—and joyfully—by immersing himself in the world of birds. Written with humility and a good dose of humour, Bell's journey is inspiring in the way he embraces a new passion with utter curiosity, and reinvents himself with remarkable resilience when life throws him a curve ball.

~ *Julia Zarankin, author of Field Notes from an Unintentional Birder*

A great read about one man's struggles and how nature heals. I am so glad that Bob found birds, not only for the healing power they gave him, but for what he has given back to birds through this book.

~ *Chris Earley, University of Guelph Arboretum Interpretive Biologist and author of Feed the Birds: Attract and Identify 196 Common North American Birds, as well as several bird field guides*

I only knew Bob Bell from running into him out in the field now and again while birding with others. He was always a friendly person with a keen love of birds. It was clear he hadn't birded for all of his life and so I'd wondered how he got into it. I've been birding since the age of 11 and I always find people's stories of how they found birding as an adult interesting to learn. A while later I became informed that he suffered from Lyme and it gave me another point of curiosity regarding Bob. Why would someone decide upon a hobby that often requires getting out and walking? My limited understanding of Lyme was that walking a lot could prove to be quite uncomfortable. So it was strange to me that Bob would take up birding, of all things. It turns out I would have all my questions answered before I even got to know Bob because of this very book you're about to enjoy. Bob's book placed me directly into his life experience; at first, it's dominated by his love of rocks, and how Lyme isolated him from that love. Then, the all-consuming Lyme melts into the background revealing his saviour, wild birds. I have known others who say birding 'saved them' but this book is the first time I've truly understood the power behind such a statement. This story will introduce you to a wonderfully kind man that took his health into his own hands and is fast becoming a great friend of mine. Enjoy.

~ *Paul Riss, Founding Partner of ROUND Agency Inc. and PRBY Art. Member & Board Director for The American Birding Association. Leading role in CBC documentary, Rare Bird Alert*

DEDICATION

This is for you, Dad.

Thanks for both instilling and nurturing my love of nature and science.

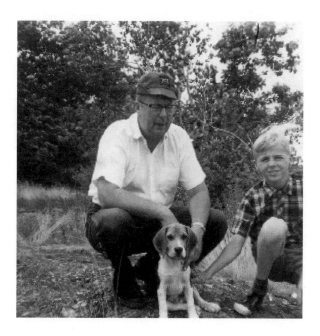

When my favourite band, Led Zeppelin, performed in concert, lead singer Robert Plant would often introduce their epic "Stairway to Heaven" as "a song of hope." My goal is that readers living with a chronic illness might find this book "a story of hope," though I hasten to add that I'm certainly not making any comparison between it and the brilliance of "Stairway to Heaven."

Alex Trebek, the longtime host of the hit TV show "Jeopardy!" and a fellow Canadian from northern Ontario, once said: "If you can't be in awe of Mother Nature, there's something wrong with you." Amen to that.

Anne Frank, in the classic "The Diary of a Young Girl": "Nature makes me feel humble and ready to face every blow with courage!"

For me, the word "birds" is an acronym for "Birding Inevitably Reduces Disease Symptoms!"

—Bob Bell

FOREWORD

Out of the Lyme Light and into the Sunlight interweaves two subjects that have dominated my life for the past nine years: Lyme disease and birding. I am honoured to have an expert on each topic write a Foreword from their perspective. The first Foreword is by Lyme specialist Dr. Kenneth Liegner, and the second by Frank Izaguirre, an editor of the American Birding Association's *Birding* magazine.

—Robert Bell

Dr. Kenneth B. Liegner, M.D., Pawling, New York
Robert C. Bell's accessible prose details his odyssey with Lyme and other tick-borne disease (e.g. babesiosis) as 'Nature' got a little 'too close' to him. He relates his frustrating obstacle-strewn path to securing a diagnosis and treatment and then finding his way 'back to the Well' – to the healing capacity of Nature.

Mr. Bell trained as a geologist and worked in mineral exploration, seeking new deposits of valuable minerals and metals in diverse geographic regions. Surely, this could have exposed him to ticks and the diseases they carry although, like many who contract Lyme disease, he had no recollection of a specific tick attachment nor of the classic Bull's eye rash which, for some 'lucky few', herald the onset of Lyme disease. Symptoms insidiously accrued including those affecting his cognitive functioning. These symptoms, in aggregate, compelled him to retire early from a challenging, high-paced career which he loved. Combined with divorce, he had to 're-invent' himself and with the help of a loving and supportive new partner forge a new life-trajectory.

A hectic globe-trotter, often without time for self-reflection, transformed himself in to an absorbed and passionate observer of those descendants of the dinosaurs: birds. He discovered that observation of these beautiful, complex and fascinating creatures conferred healing. Whether merely watching from the ease and comfort of the living room picture-window of his new forest-ensconced home or taking afield, camera and/or binocular bedecked, solo or with birding companions to diverse habitats, his avian subjects enabled him to shift his attention from physical symptoms of illness to joyful passion observing Nature. This enabled him to often overcome, if not completely eliminate, symptoms that had previously limited his functioning. Along the way, his life was enriched by deep friendships with others who shared his passion for birds and the Natural World.

His book is graced with excellent quality photographs of some of his bird-subjects including many elusive warblers and also provides readers with links to pertinent birding resources and references.

Whether or not readers suffer from Lyme disease or other chronic illnesses, Mr. Bell's volume enriches the reader and inspires one to overcome obstacles and to realize there are many paths to Wellness.

> —*Dr. Kenneth Liegner is a Board-Certified Internist with additional training in Pathology and Critical Care Medicine, practicing in Pawling, New York. He has been actively involved in diagnosis and treatment of Lyme disease and related disorders since 1988. Dr. Liegner has published numerous articles on Lyme disease and has presented at national and international conferences on the topic. He is on the staff of Northern Westchester Hospital Center in Mount Kisco, New York and the Sharon Hospital in Sharon, Connecticut.*

Frank Izaguirre, Pittsburgh, Pennsylvania

On an intuitive level, birders know that birding is good for our health: it gets us outside, often involves exercise, and is fun. But some birders know on an even deeper level that birding is good for health, because in times of serious illness and personal struggle, birding can be a lifeline.

Robert Bell's remarkable *Out of the Lyme Light and Into the Sunlight* tells the story of one such birder with grace, honesty, and moving prose. Readers learn of Bell's struggle to receive an accurate diagnosis for Lyme disease, the intense stress of navigating the healthcare system, and the crippling and life-altering pain. We learn also of Bell's resilience in the face of these challenges, and, most joyfully, of his discovery of birding as an elixir of pain relief and purpose when times were toughest.

Although I have not suffered from Lyme disease, as a cancer survivor I can candidly say that I saw myself in Bell's experience with long-term illness: the pain, the despair, the frustration. And I can also say that I saw myself in Bell's enthusiastic endorsement of birding as a form of therapy. Although I had already been a birder for many years before I was first diagnosed with colon cancer at the age of 26, I too found birding to be a vital lifeline as what had once been my life crumbled before me, and as I braced for and recovered from major surgery.

So it was again, when two years later, I learned that the cancer had metastasized, and I had to cancel my wedding and abandon my career to prepare for aggressive chemotherapy and another surgery. Yet again, three years later, when the cancer was once more detected—amid the surgery, recovery, brutal chemo, and disintegration of what had been my normal life—birds and birding were there. It is almost impossible for me to imagine going through those awful things without the birds.

Out of the Lyme Light and Into the Sunlight joins the growing literature of books about both birding and well-being, as more individuals tell their own tales of struggle and how birding sustained them through tremendously challenging times. Bell's book is exceptional in that not only does he tell his own compelling story, he also directly lists many resources for readers still learning about birding, both in the main story and in various thoughtful appendices. Wellness resources are also listed.

I believe this book will help people: people with Lyme disease, people with other serious illnesses, and people who are scared as they navigate the challenges of self-advocacy in medicine. It will help because sick people often feel like they are suffering alone, but they aren't really alone—they're just isolated from others enduring similar experiences.

Robert Bell's brave book helps fix that by connecting people. Those who have had or are having similar experiences may feel less alone, and perhaps avoid some of the difficulties he faced. In his own words, Bell writes: "Birding saved my life." As readers, we are fortunate this is the case, because Bell has written something wonderful that may in turn help save the lives of others. At the core of Bell's book is the sincere belief that not only can birds help heal, but also that we can all help heal each other. May we all be reminded of this truth whenever we feel the joy of birding.

—*Frank Izaguirre is co-editor of* Birding *magazine and also reviews editor for* Birding. *He is also a doctoral candidate in English at West Virginia University, where he is dissertating on how field guides have influenced environmental thinking.*

TABLE OF CONTENTS

PREFACE

In August 2013, my older sister, Barb, was about to turn 60 and had recently retired. She had always dreamed of touring Africa but never had the opportunity. As a geologist, I had made innumerable business trips to southern Africa and at that time was overseeing copper exploration programs in Namibia. With Barb's retirement and milestone birthday coming up, I had a double reason to help make her dream come true.

During the last two weeks of August 2013 we toured South Africa, Botswana, Zambia, and Namibia. We spent a few days in cabins on the Zambezi River close to Victoria Falls, listening to hippos snorting away at night. I recollect sustaining a number of insect bites during our stay; at the time I thought: *Better a bug than a hippo chomping on me.*

A week or so after returning home, I awoke in the middle of the night drenched in sweat, with uncontrollable cold chills and a very high fever. *Bloody hell,* I thought, to borrow a phrase commonly used by my Australian colleagues. I had contracted dengue fever a few years earlier, while working in the Amazon in Brazil, and I clearly remembered the infectious disease doctor wagging his finger at me, warning me to not ever catch it again. He had lectured me that a second infection could become hemorrhagic and potentially be fatal. What I was experiencing after our trip to Africa was identical to my first symptoms of "breakbone fever," as dengue is commonly called. "Here I go again," I thought.

I did not foresee the life-altering path that I was about to travel down. Here I go, indeed—down the rabbit hole that is Lyme disease, its diagnosis (or lack thereof), and treatment. As my dad was fond of saying, I didn't know the half of it.

1. INTRODUCTION

I am, or more accurately, *was*, a mineral exploration geologist. At some point in my global travels I apparently encountered a Lyme-infected tick or insect of some sort that gave me Lyme disease. My fulfilling, challenging occupation—my life-long passion for being paid to spend much of my time outdoors on a literal treasure hunt—came to a sudden halt. However, as one door closed, another opened. The old adage that one man's crisis is another's opportunity came true for me. I discovered a new passion: birding, one that got my mind off of my faltering, aching body. Coincidentally, my new passion of birding, like mineral exploration, is also a treasure hunt: you never know what gem you might find hidden in the trees, brambles, or reeds. My goal with this story is to instill hope and optimism in fellow Lyme-sufferers and other people who have to deal with chronic pain and fatigue. My intent is to demonstrate that birding can be an effective form of therapy for almost anyone who suffers from long-term pain.

I had always known that "Little Bobby's Big Adventures," as my then ten-year-old daughter had dubbed my career, brought more than its fair share of risks. I had survived a helicopter crash; a lightning strike that missed me by about ten metres; some incredibly unsanitary or unconventional (to a Canadian) food, and food poisoning; several earthquakes; dengue fever; parasitic infections and malarial-like symptoms; a float plane running out of fuel mid-air and another landing on a lake in the dark as I hung out the door to give the pilot estimates of our altitude and talk him down; and a trigger-happy guard at a gold mine in Brazil pointing an assault rifle at my head. Assuming the fever I sustained on the return from my African trip with Barb was another potential bout of dengue fever, I thought to myself: *No little insect bite will be the end of the line for me.* This new bout of fever, cold chills, and general malaise lasted for three days and then faded away on its own. Knowing that the dengue fever I had previously experienced had lasted about a week, I relaxed and forgot all about it.

Starting roughly six weeks later, every morning when I awoke, the arm on the side I'd been sleeping on stayed "asleep," with feelings of numbness and a pins-and-needles sensation. It took a minute or so to get rid of the painful tingles. Although this was something new and unusual, I would quickly forget about it as I got on with my busy days.

Within a week or so, however, the tops of my feet started burning and tingling, hurting so badly that when lying in bed I couldn't let them touch each other. Even wearing socks hurt. These bizarre sensations became my new normal and persisted, day after day. A few weeks later, I experienced a strange new sensation—my muscles, particularly in the triceps and biceps of one arm, began to throb in a deep, painful way. I couldn't sleep on that arm for very long before the pain became unbearable, and I had to continuously flip from side to side, resulting in very poor, non-restorative sleep. The muscle pain was so intense that I could not hold a phone to my ear for more than a minute or two; I had to use the hands-free speaker. But the weirdness was just beginning. That arm would stop aching, but then a few days later the muscles in my upper back would become sore, and soon the pain would migrate to the other arm, then my lower back, and on and on. My girlfriend, Irina, who is a dentist with general medical training, warned me that if I complained to a doctor that I had migratory muscle pain, they'd think I was crazy. How right Irina was; she had unintentionally foreshadowed my looming battle with our conventional medical system, while at the same time she had unknowingly identified one of the signature symptoms of Lyme disease.

A benign tremor that runs in our family suddenly became a Parkinson's-like shake in my hands. I developed crepitus, a very loud *snap, crackle and pop* type of cracking in my wrist joints; I could perform wrist-cracking percussion practically on demand. This sound, offensive to many of my friends, then spread into my finger joints and my ankles. I figured crepitus was a very appropriate word, given that I felt like I was becoming decrepit!

For the first time in my life, I was constantly aware of my body. This all-consuming awareness made me realize that when we are healthy, we are essentially, and thankfully, unaware of our bodies.

I started feeling weaker, and it became a chore to walk. Irina and I would go for a walk, but I would be exhausted after only several hundred metres; she would have to support me and push me from behind to propel me forward if there was even the slightest incline. I quickly reached the point that I required a cane for support and stability. An overwhelming fatigue would typically kick in between about noon and 2 p.m. I would go to work in the morning, "hit the wall" around noon, and have to head home for a one- to two-hour nap. Up till then, I had never been able to sleep in the daytime, except for when I was truly sick with something such as the flu. Now, I required a nap every day, and I often felt so groggy after awakening from these naps that the rest of the day was shot.

Although I was extremely concerned, not knowing what mysterious ailment was afflicting me, I did not tell anyone other than my day-to-day business colleagues and Terry MacGibbon, the chairman of the board of directors for the mineral exploration and development company where I served as CEO. It had become increasingly hard to hide my severe tremor, my need to urinate about every two hours, and my obvious discomfort, exhibited by grimaces of pain as I constantly adjusted my sitting position during meetings. I was running out of excuses as to why I was constantly leaving work early. I recall saying to Terry, "There's something strange going on with me, I think neurologically." I held out my arm to show him my hand trembling uncontrollably.

Over the Christmas holidays in 2013, I arranged a visit with a psychically gifted friend who has the uncanny ability to "know things"—a gift about which, as a scientist, I was highly skeptical. I had always enjoyed catching up with her as a friend; however, this time I was curious to hear what she might have to say about my physical condition. I deliberately didn't mention anything about my symptoms to her ahead of time, so as not to "lead the witness." I heard her knock on the door, and as soon as I anxiously opened it, she said, "OK, spill it. What's going on with your health?" It is important to point out that I did not look sick; in fact, a common frustration for Lyme victims is when well-meaning friends say, "Well, you *look* good." The unspoken implication is that it's all in your head, or that it can't be that bad if you look so good. My anxiety dissipated as I realized that her knowing instantly that something was wrong with me meant that I wasn't crazy and imagining it. Immediately after my knee-jerk reaction of initial relief, my second thought was, "Wait, is there actually something real about psychic abilities?" I admit that this will not be very convincing for many readers, but for me, this suddenly provided one good reason to be a little less skeptical of this friend's psychic abilities. But what was "it" that was happening to me? After I described my symptoms, she insisted I see a doctor as soon as possible. I explained that I had a very thorough annual physical checkup booked for March, three months away. She insisted that I reschedule it to the earliest possible date, which of course made me anxious once again! She went on to say that whatever was wrong was not going to kill me, but the sooner it was diagnosed and treated, the better my odds would be of recovery. Again, a very prescient comment about Lyme, which can be highly curable when treated promptly. Based on her insistence, I rescheduled the appointment to early January, just a couple of weeks away.

2. ABOUT ME: BACKGROUND AND ADVENTURES

I lived a busy, energetic, and fulfilling life before Lyme. If you'd like to know what that looked like, here's my background. If you don't, feel free to skip this chapter. I'm lucky that once again my life has become busy, energetic, and fulfilling, in a totally different way; however, it has been quite a journey into my darkest days with Lyme and out again.

I grew up in Sault Ste. Marie, Ontario, Canada (commonly known as the "Soo"), a small city in Northern Ontario situated on the locks connecting two of the Great Lakes, Lake Superior and Lake Huron. My late father, Thomas Arthur Bell, was a high school vice-principal and science teacher with a Bachelor of Science degree in agriculture. He had a vast knowledge of botany, biology, chemistry, physics, astronomy, and nature in general. Dad instilled in me a passion and thirst for reading, knowledge, nature, and science that has made me who I am and has shaped my life, my interests, and my career. We had a cottage on Bright Lake, located 100 kilometres east of the Soo. Every weekend from early May until Thanksgiving was spent at the cottage, and Dad, being a teacher, had the summer off, so we were also there for the entire months of July and August. All that time spent there cemented a lifetime love of the outdoors and the natural world.

My father got me started on a rock and mineral collection and helped me identify all of the various treasures I found and brought home. I believe my career as a geologist was destined when I was a toddler playing in a sandbox in the small Northern Ontario town of New Liskeard, where I was born in the late 1950s. My mother claimed that she could leave Bobby in the sandbox for hours with no worries that he would roam; apparently, I just sat there fascinated by the sand.

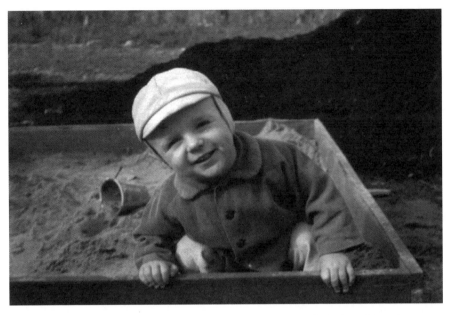

Geologist in training, about 1959

As a child I built and organized numerous collections, including stamps and insects, especially butterflies and moths. My new love of seeing as many bird species as possible and collecting and organizing bird photos is a natural fit with this life-long interest in nature and probably obsessive-compulsive desire to collect and organize. I spent every winter Saturday morning with my paternal grandfather, who would allow me to go through a huge box of duplicate stamps from his collection and keep about a dozen or so. I recall how, after buying a two-volume global stamp album, I would run home daily after school in Grade 9 so that I could work on it, putting stickers of flags for each country in the albums, and finding the correct pages and spots to place the stamps passed on from my Grandpa. Thus, my love and knowledge of geography was sparked. Little did I know that someday I would be lucky enough to have a career that would take me to many of these far-off, exotic places that I could only dream about during those formative years. Nor did I know that my childhood passions for nature and science were setting the stage for a career in earth science.

Growing up in the era of "moon shots," I became deeply interested in astronomy and space. I vividly remember that fateful day in July 1969, at the age of 12, watching in awe on my maternal grandparents' black-and-white television in Palmerston, Ontario, the grainy images of Neil Armstrong descending the Eagle's ladder to the surface of the moon. I would run outside to look up at the moon, run back to the TV, and back outside. Although this didn't inspire me to become an astronaut, it did lead to my parents getting me a telescope, powerful enough to see the four Galilean moons of Jupiter, the rings of Saturn, and the polar caps on Mars. It was in constant use during our summers at camp, where the skies were void of light pollution and therefore excellent for star-gazing.

When I started at the University of Western Ontario (now Western University) in London, Ontario, I intended to obtain a Bachelor of Chemistry degree, then use that as a springboard to apply to medical school. I cruised through my first-year general science courses, then majored in chemistry starting in my second year. However, I was no match for the Organic Chemistry course. By the time I realized that I would never pass it, it was November and too late to change majors. I just coasted through the rest of my second year, passing all of my courses except "Orgo."

Since getting into medical school wasn't in the cards, I decided the life of a geologist would be exciting and a good fit for me, with my rock and mineral collection and love of the outdoors, nature, and science (to say nothing of all that experience in my sandbox). Thus, in my third year at university I entered second-year geology and found myself on the "five-year plan" to getting my four-year bachelor's degree. I found that I did less work and studying in geology than I did in chemistry, but my marks were twenty percent higher. I graduated in April 1980 with an Honours Bachelor of Science in Geology. After graduation, I took a summer mineral exploration job in British Columbia with Canadian mining giant Inco Ltd (now Vale Canada Ltd), and then joined them permanently in January 1981, following a brief, aborted effort to do a geology doctorate at the University of Melbourne in Australia.

Not long after I joined Inco, I bought a house in Sudbury, Ontario, the home of the majority of Inco's copper-nickel mines. I thought having a roommate would be helpful, not only in meeting my mortgage payments but by ensuring that someone would be home to keep an eye on the house while I was away working for extended periods of time. My sister Barb suggested her friend Leslie, who had just returned from the United States, where she had completed a master's in education, and needed a place to stay. It wasn't long before I married my roommate! We had two beautiful children, Candace and Trevor, who in their teen years began to accompany me on various international trips. After thirty years of marriage, Leslie and I divorced in 2012.

I remained at Inco for twenty-seven years, ultimately serving as Director of International Exploration. I quit in 2007 after Inco was taken over by Vale, a Brazilian company, and the business culture changed too drastically for me. This was just three years shy of earning a full pension, and for leaving early I lost sixty percent of it, even though I was ninety percent of the way there.

Annoyingly, geologists are not often recognized as professionals; in fact, we are openly mocked, as anyone who has watched the television show *The Big Bang Theory* knows. The character Sheldon referred to geologists as "the dirt people" and frequently ranted that "geology is not a real science!" I figure geology is the Rodney Dangerfield of sciences—it gets no respect.

When Ontario finally introduced professional registration for geoscientists, giving us self-regulating professional status similar to lawyers, doctors, dentists, and engineers, my younger sister, Brenda, gave me the following pin. No mocking or sarcasm intended, of course.

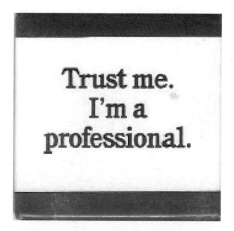

Respect at last. (BUTR-773815©RPP, Inc.)

The discovery of a mineral deposit large and rich enough to ultimately be mined is a rare event. I regret to say that I am among the majority of geologists who have never experienced the thrill of such an event, although I have been involved in several exciting mineral discoveries that weren't quite the right scale to be economically exploited. Given the excitement I felt from those, I can only imagine how explorationists feel when they make a world-class discovery, an ore body worth billions of dollars that might employ up to several generations of miners, and around which an entire town might be established. This thrill of the treasure hunt is what motivates geologists to literally leave no stone unturned. It is with great delight that I can say I now get that same feeling of exhilaration, excitement, and jubilation when I see a rare bird, or a bird that is new to me, and when I do, I feel like the healthiest person on the planet.

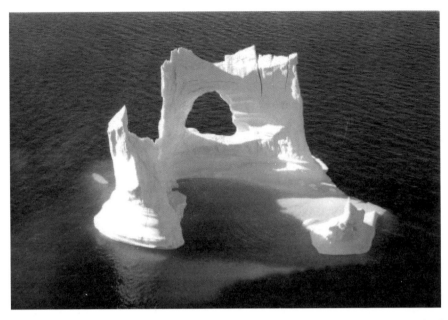

Ice cathedral off the coast of Greenland

My career provided me opportunities to visit many exotic locales. One of my favorite environments in the world is the Arctic. I've been lucky to experience 24-hour daylight in the Canadian Arctic, Greenland, Iceland, and the Norbotten district of northern Sweden. I think one of the most breathtaking sights I have ever seen was this iceberg, which I photographed from a helicopter off the west coast of Greenland. Geologists always put a scale bar in photos they take of rocks, so one can tell if the subject is a small hand sample or a huge outcrop. If I didn't happen to have an actual map scale with me when geologic mapping, I'd use a quarter, which inevitably led to my mother questioning why I kept taking photos of money. Unfortunately, this photo doesn't have a boat or some other object to serve as a scale bar to convey the majestic size of the iceberg; that hole at the top was large enough to fly the helicopter through, if one was that daring (or reckless).

Far from the Arctic, I have stood on the equator in both Indonesia and Ecuador; it is a strange thing to cast no shadow, or a very tiny one only immediately below you at noon, when the sun is directly overhead. Likewise, it is funny to see satellite dishes lying almost flat on their backs, pointing straight up, unlike in Canada where because of our high latitude they are tipped close to vertical in order to be in contact with the satellites stationed above the earth's equator.

My travels have allowed me to see many world-famous sights, including the Great Wall of China, Red Square in Moscow, the Hermitage in St. Petersburg, the Atacama Desert of Chile, Machu Picchu in Peru, the Borobudur Hindu temple in Java, Indonesia, Uluru (Ayers Rock) in Australia, Iguaçu Falls on the border of Argentina and Brazil, the spectacular red sand dunes at Sossusvlei, Namibia, and the Christian caves at Cappadocia, Turkey. Although I previously mentioned surviving a helicopter crash, I have thoroughly enjoyed helicopter flights in the high Andes of Peru, over Victoria Falls in Africa, over lava flows on the Big Island of Hawaii, and the highlands of Irian Jaya, Indonesia (now West Papua).

I contracted the parasite Cryptosporidium in Peru, and as mentioned in the preface, I caught dengue fever in the Amazon basin of Brazil. With all of this international travel, I have been exposed to many different terrains and environments, including whatever infectious diseases might be carried by various insects or ticks there. I am not aware of ever getting a tick bite, which is not uncommon in people with Lyme disease. This is not surprising, as even the pinhead-sized nymphs are believed to be potentially infectious.

My doctor told me on more than one occasion that my extensive travel was killing me. It turns out that statement was a little too prophetic to be comfortable, but for a different reason. His concern was my constant state of jet lag; he claimed that it really is true that you need a day per time zone passed through to fully recover. I can remember once flying from Toronto, Canada, to Brisbane, Australia, for a one-and-a-half-day meeting and being back home within five days of leaving, only to head off to South America a few days later. At that time Brisbane was fifteen hours ahead of Toronto, so I did not have the luxury of thirty days to recover from that journey.

I have flown close to three million miles, the equivalent of six round trips to the moon, or 120 times around the world, including thirty trips to Australia and forty-five to Brazil. Mind you, this is par for the course for the mining business. One winter, I was waiting to board an Air Canada flight to return from the Canadian bank BMO's annual mining investment conference in Florida; when they announced pre-boarding for Elite and Super Elite frequent-flyer members, about three-quarters of the passengers in the departure lounge stood up.

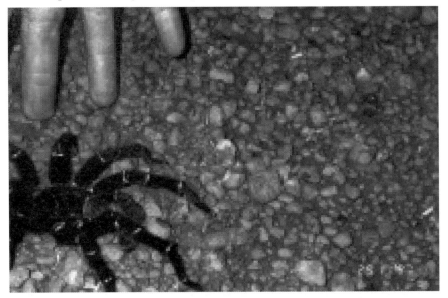

One of many hazards of conducting mineral exploration

In hindsight, I don't know how I managed all the travel, and I don't miss it in the least. Lots of friends and family used to express jealousy, asking if they could stow away in my suitcase. I always replied, "Travel is only exotic and appealing to those who don't travel." These were not vacations planned at convenient times; they were business trips, and one followed the next relentlessly. If I started an exploration project in a new country, after a few trips with an adventurous spirit, the novelty would quickly wear thin. Travel would then simply become stressful, especially post-9/11, and particularly if I had to travel to or transit through the United States, where passport control could be intimidating, to say the least.

I have had innumerable encounters with wildlife, and not just ticks and tiny insects. On a trip to the wild west of Brazil, we were a bit late getting back to our hotel and broke our safety rules by driving in the dark. In the truck headlights you could see large black objects on the road. When we stopped to investigate, we could hear the gravel crunching beneath the feet of the black objects; they were huge tarantulas! I wanted to take a photo of one, and as discussed previously, needed something for scale in order to demonstrate its true size. Our chief geologist, Dave, volunteered his hand as a scale, and I attempted to take the photo. In the dark I had a hard time seeing where to aim my camera, so you will see that my photo is off-centre. Eventually, my flash went off. The tarantula jumped about three feet straight up. Dave jumped about five feet straight up.

I've had several encounters with much larger animals, in particular bears. In the spring of 1986, when I was working with Inco, a geological technician, Cesar, and I established a drive-in tent camp on a project just west of Gogama, north of Sudbury, Ontario. We were plagued by black bears; they were only recently out of hibernation, so were scruffy, scrawny, and starving. The spring bear hunt was on, and there were bear hunters camped just down the road from us. How sporting to put out rotting, maggoty meat and wait for a starving bear to show up so you can shoot him. They were having no luck, probably because the bears were all hanging out at our camp. We managed to fend the bears off most nights by banging on pots and pans, but as the days went by, we could see they were becoming a little more aggressive. One evening, the two of us were sleeping on our cots in our tent when Cesar let out a scream. I hit the dirt wide awake, grabbing our rifle just in case. It turned out that Cesar had run a wire from our high frequency radio cable and wrapped it around his transistor radio in order to boost its reception. The wire ran from the coaxial cable coming off the antennae into our tent, under his bed, and under the flap of a cardboard box on which his radio was sitting. A bear had gone by within feet of our tent, got tangled in the wire, and when he pulled away, Cesar's cot actually rocked, hence the scream.

We sat up and waited, but things went quiet. After going back to bed, at one point I realized there was a lump in the tent wall next to my head—it was the bear sniffing me through the canvas. We got up again, and eventually the bear was making motions to come in through the front door. We threw a lit Coleman lantern out, which almost started a fire but didn't startle the bear.

Eventually the bear made a charge for the front of the door. Unfortunately, we had to shoot him dead on the doorstop. It was not that he was intruding on our space; we had set up camp on his turf and he didn't deserve to die for that. My life-long love of nature is clearly a double-edged sword; there is always potential danger lurking just beneath the surface, whether it is a huge black bear or a pinhead-sized tick nymph.

My travels also permitted me to experience numerous cultures around the world. I was lucky to visit an Inco project in Irian Jaya (West Papua) on the island of New Guinea, which Indonesia shares with Papua New Guinea. It is probably the last, most remote and difficult to access, pre-industrial place on the planet. A sheer mountain range forms a spine down the centre of the island; one peak has a glacier even though it is close to the equator (or had; it was rapidly receding in 1996). One of my most surreal experiences was walking into the local hotel where we were staying. I passed a fellow standing at the doorway selling crafts, buck naked except for a "koteka" (a penis gourd to provide modesty), pig tusks through his nostrils, and a cassowary-feather headdress. Two steps later, I was in the lobby of the hotel where a TV was playing a music video by the rock band U2. Like Neil Armstrong's "That's one small step for man, one giant leap for mankind," that seemed like a 10,000-year leap in time!

Similarly, in northern Namibia resides a group of indigenous people called the Himba. The women go topless and cover their bodies in a mixture of butter fat and red ochre; their sense of modesty is protected by wearing silver ankle bracelets. I happened to be in a local grocery store lineup, with a young Himba woman behind me, dressed traditionally and texting on her cell phone. The juxtaposition of her ancient customs and modern technology brought a cognitive dissonance that was startling, to say the least. Although I believe the red ochre is meant to protect their skin from the sun, I can't help but wonder if it isn't also to protect against infectious insects. After all, those koteka-sporting people in Irian Jaya smelled a bit "ripe," thanks to their custom of coating themselves in pig grease to ward off disease-carrying insects.

My son Trevor accompanied me on a business trip to Namibia in 2011. We took a side trip to Livingstone, Zambia, and from there traveled to Chobe National Park in Botswana. This requires a ferry to cross the river border. Numerous vendors capitalize on the captive audience of tourists waiting for the ferry. A fellow came along peddling copper bracelets. Trevor explained he had no cash, only a Canadian Tire bill that he'd been using as a bookmark. Even though Trevor was honest enough to explain that Canadian Tire money was not real currency and only valid in the Canadian hardware chain, the vendor didn't care. He enthusiastically traded a bracelet for it, telling us how happy he was to have something from Canada. On another day, near Victoria Falls, Trevor was bartering with a vendor for three wooden carvings. Although they had settled on a fair price, the vendor begged him to include his ankle socks, stating "My wife would be so proud." Off came the socks and Trevor got his carvings. Trev took the photo of me, when we were on a cruise down the Zambezi River watching hippopotamus, crocodiles, and elephants. Note I'm wearing a Monty Python shirt that says, "I'm not dead yet." If I had a crystal ball, I'd have known that in a few short years, immediately after another trip to that same location in Africa, I was going to need to wear that shirt just to perk myself up.

As much as I've been privileged to see many exotic places in the world, the most rewarding aspect has been making friends in numerous countries, from Japan, Australia, and Turkey, to Indonesia, Namibia, Brazil, Peru, Ecuador, and many more. I have learned just enough of a number of foreign languages to be dangerous. One thing I've found worldwide is that what is important is not the degree of your proficiency in someone's language, but rather, your effort. Learning the basics of hi and goodbye, please and thank you is almost universally rewarded with a warm smile.

For anyone who might be interesting in reading more about adventures in mineral exploration and development, please see Appendix C, where I've given a brief summary of four books I recommend on this subject.

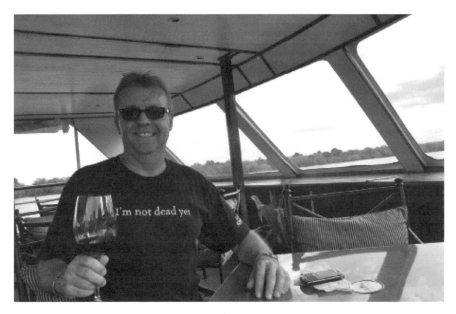

Not dead yet!

I have gone into a fair bit of detail on my career and travel adventures with the intent of demonstrating that I had a pretty active, busy, go-go-go career and lifestyle that I loved. Lyme disease brought it to a screeching halt.

3. THE FRUSTRATION BEGINS

My annual medical in early January 2014 was the start of a long, frustrating road; I learned very quickly that to navigate through the medical system you have to become your own advocate. My highly rated, highly qualified doctor dismissed the "asleep" sensation in my arms as simply due to the position of my sleep. I remember thinking, "REALLY? I'm almost 57 years old—I do have a bit of experience sleeping. That's the best you've got?" He did, however, refer me to a rheumatologist. I told her before she even examined me that I thought I was wasting her time, that I believed I needed to see a neurologist. She quickly determined that my symptoms did not indicate arthritis which might have resulted in a pinched nerve, and also agreed that I needed to see a neurologist. I went back to the clinic and obtained a referral to a neurologist. All of this time, the clock was ticking, and I kept remembering the emphatic warning from my clairvoyant friend to not waste time. As I mentioned previously, Lyme is usually highly curable if treated promptly.

Awaiting the neurologist appointment, I found myself walking into furniture and clunking dishes into the kitchen cupboard doorframes to the point of breaking a few. It seemed my sense of where my body was in space was off. You don't realize how effective your brain is at mapping your spatial position in three dimensions until that function stops working properly. Increasingly, I was worried that I was developing multiple sclerosis (MS) or amyotrophic lateral sclerosis (ALS), commonly known as Lou Gehrig's disease or motor neuron disease. As I would eventually learn, Lyme is called "the great imitator" because its symptoms mirror those of a number of neurological diseases, including MS, ALS, and Parkinson's.

What the Lyme doctors euphemistically call "brain fog" started. I got to the point that I could not count out a couple of dollars in change to buy a newspaper, which left me extremely frustrated and embarrassed. Worse, I felt that I was beginning to lose control of my emotions. The least bit of incompetence in a store clerk would send me into a rage. At one point, I was in a meeting with the mines minister of a country where my company was working to develop a gold mine. We had simultaneous translation between Spanish and English. The translator was very good; he even imitated tone of voice when something was emphasized. I knew I had a real problem when I could hear the translator shouting my words at the mines minister in Spanish! Not a way to win friends and influence people.

The neurologist put me through extensive testing, including an MRI. He also gave me two types of rather unpleasant nerve conduction tests, during which I was given electric shocks and the response time for the signal to travel along my nerves or muscles was recorded. When all the test results were in, the neurologist literally washed his hands of me, dismissing me with a bit of a smirk, "I'm sorry, but you do *not* have a neurological disease." Since I apparently didn't have a neurological disease, even though I had plenty of neurological symptoms, he was done with me, without any concern about what *was* causing my problems.

However, the neurologist did ask me a key question that set me to thinking: "Have you had any recent infections or fevers?" He said that they could occasionally trigger neurological problems. I suddenly remembered the fever and chills I had shortly after my African trip, and about a month prior to the onset of strange symptoms such as burning, tingling, and pins-and-needles and "asleep" sensations. This reminded me that I had feared a recurrence of dengue fever, which in turn got me thinking of insect-borne diseases. I knew I had been bitten by unknown insects multiple times during our two-week journey through Africa. I was later told by my Lyme specialist in upstate New York that Lyme can remain dormant in your body for years, before being activated by a subsequent infection. Either that fever was the initial onset of me contracting Lyme disease on my African travels, or, given my extensive travel history and exposure to potential disease vectors all over the world, it was possibly just a random infection that triggered latent Lyme which I had been unwittingly harboring.

Having been dismissed by the neurologist, I returned to the medical clinic to request a referral to an infectious disease expert. Being your own health care advocate is not easy when you're emotionally and physically unwell; if you don't push, the system is happy to ignore symptoms it can't explain. I got a referral and was sent to be tested for malaria and chikungunya (both mosquito-born, the former a parasite and the latter a viral infection), and, unbeknownst to me, syphilis. I was surprised to find out at the follow-up appointment that I had been tested for it; I had no idea that late-stage syphilis can present some of the neurological abnormalities I was experiencing. Interestingly, the bacterium that causes syphilis, like the Lyme bacterium, is screw-shaped, called a spirochete. My understanding is that is why a classic Lyme symptom is migratory muscle pain—the spirochetes are literally corkscrewing their way through your muscles. Happily, I was told that I did not have any of those diseases; unhappily, I had reached a dead end.

Hearing I was unwell, my good friend Sara Kernan dropped by my condo one evening for a visit. While I was describing my symptoms to Sara and my frustration at the lack of a diagnosis, I could see that my story had triggered something in her mind. She interrupted me to say that I should be tested for Lyme; stating that my symptoms sounded very familiar to those presented by her friend Pierrette Donaghy. As it turns out, Pierrette isn't Sara's only friend with Lyme! Not only did Sara open my eyes to a possibility I hadn't considered, she connected me with Pierrette. As a result, I gained a new friend who was highly knowledgeable about Lyme, understanding about what I was going through, and empathetic to my plight.

Shortly after that, I had a coffee with Jamile Cruz, a Brazilian friend who works as a mining engineer based in Toronto. Like me, Jamile's work requires extensive travel that exposes her to numerous food-borne pathogens. She had been looking for a long time for a diagnosis and treatment that would explain and alleviate her stomach pains. She heard about a complementary health practitioner who specialized in electrodermal testing for various types of infections. He ran his tests and told her what he thought was causing her particular health issue. His diagnosis was later confirmed by conventional medical testing. Jamile, being aware of and concerned about my mysterious ailments, thought that I should make an appointment. She warned me that this fellow was a slightly eccentric character but recommended that I give him a chance.

Since I was growing increasingly frustrated with conventional medicine, I booked an appointment at the complementary practitioner's midtown Toronto office in late June 2014. He had me hold a metal rod that he set to vibrating at various frequencies, while my feet rested on metal plates. By measuring some sort of energy balance, his computer software then supposedly could identify the infectious agent or agents. It all seemed bizarre, but at this point I was desperate to know what was going wrong with my body and my mind. In some ways, his procedure is an analogue to a Rife machine, which I will discuss later in Chapter 14. This was now eight months since the onset of my mysterious symptoms and six months since my friend implored me to get on with a medical treatment as soon as possible. The practitioner ran frequencies for 240 parasites, bacteria, and viruses. Out of these, I apparently responded to only six, all of which were Lyme strains or typical Lyme co-infections. "It's a spear-rocket, mate!" he loudly proclaimed, mispronouncing spirochete ("spy-row-keet").

Having an unconventional "diagnosis" of Lyme disease in hand, I returned to the conventional medical system. Even though I thought I was fully prepared for the skepticism and eye-rolling to come, it turned out I wasn't. At this point, my adventures and frustration were about to really take off.

4. LYME DIAGNOSIS AND TREATMENT

I returned to the medical clinic and requested a blood test for Lyme disease. My doctor immediately responded, "Well, where or how could you have ever been exposed to a tick?"—as if that was so rare and unlikely that he didn't want to even consider it. I told him I was a geologist and had worked all over the world. He "harrumphed" and reluctantly agreed to administer the ELISA blood test. ELISA is an acronym for "enzyme-linked immunosorbent assay"; it does not detect the Lyme bacterium directly, but rather is used to determine if you have antibodies against it. Lyme blood tests are two-tiered; the ELISA is administered first, and if positive or indeterminate, then a second blood test called the Western Blot test is performed to confirm the diagnosis. The tests might not be positive during the early stage of Lyme disease if the body has not had time to produce detectable antibodies. This means there is a good chance you could easily get false negative results, even though you do have Lyme. Furthermore, my understanding is that ELISA apparently only tests for antibodies of a limited number of the several hundred strains of the Lyme bacteria. This would also contribute to a high rate of false negative responses. The Global Lyme Alliance states that the ELISA test is falsely negative nearly 50% of the time. My results, naturally, were negative on the ELISA test and as a result, according to my doctor, I did not have Lyme disease and was therefore denied the slightly more definitive Western Blot test. If I had been "lucky" enough to be positive on the ELISA test, I would have been eligible for the Western Blot test.

The frustrating part to me was that, although my doctor was satisfied that I did not have Lyme disease based on the bloodwork, he was ignoring all of my symptoms and didn't seem interested in trying to explain them. History was repeating itself; this was just like the neurologist dismissing me with no explanation for my neurological problems. Knowing that the blood test I had been administered for Lyme was considered untrustworthy, I wasn't about to give up. I researched and found that there was a state-of-the-art Lyme testing laboratory in Palo Alto, California, part of "Silicon Valley," called IGeneX. Since no Canadian doctor would provide a bloodwork requisition order for an American lab, I sought out a Lyme-literate naturopath who set me up with the appropriate requisition form and with a courier package to have the bloodwork sent to them.

While I awaited the results of the IGeneX test, I went under the care of the naturopath. I spent thousands of dollars on naturopathic care, because that was the only treatment available to me. These expenditures included hundreds of dollars a month for bloodwork, various supplements and herbal remedies, as well as "infusion therapy." This involved a twice-weekly intravenous drip in the late summer and autumn of 2014, a cocktail comprised of glutathione and other antioxidants. None of these alleviated my symptoms.

The IGeneX results confirmed the presence of a high number of Lyme antibodies. When I returned to the doctor at the local clinic with my new test results in hand, his condescending comment to me was, "Of course you're positive; they want your business." Unfortunately, this dismissive attitude is rampant throughout the medical system, yet it is ignorant of the facts and just plain wrong. IGeneX has no ulterior financial motive to find one positive or negative; it is solely a diagnostic lab. To quote Yogi Berra, this was "déjà vu all over again." I now had a second Lyme disease diagnosis in hand, yet conventional medicine considered it to be no more technically credible than the first one. However, the medical system could provide no explanation for my twenty or so increasingly severe symptoms and didn't seem interested in finding out their cause. I have previously described major symptoms such as fatigue, migratory muscle pain, peripheral neuropathy, and the audible joint-cracking crepitus. However, Lyme can also present a smorgasbord of seemingly unrelated, strange symptoms, including cognitive impairment and emotional instability.

I developed random muscle twitches, typically in my arms. I could watch a muscle visibly twitch away, pulsating like a heart beat, once every second or two for up to several minutes. Although already hard of hearing with fairly loud ringing in my ears, I now had roaring tinnitus, much louder and more debilitating than prior to my infection. Several times a week, I'd have heart palpitations. They felt like they went on forever but probably were no more than five to ten seconds. I had to urinate frequently, which meant my sleep was extremely disrupted, since I had to get up four or five times a night. I joked that my thermostat was broken, as I ran inordinately hot. I would sweat profusely for no reason, particularly in any social situation, which triggered debilitating anxiety. If I had to talk for very long, my voice would get extremely hoarse and raspy. If I had to climb even the slightest incline, never mind a hill, or a short flight of steps, I was out of breath and my legs turned to rubbery mush. I would often lose my balance and have to do a quick stutter step to regain it. I continued to walk into furniture, hard enough to leave large, ugly bruises. My wrists became so weak that I could barely write. This meant my signature totally changed, to the point that at work we discussed whether I'd need to give our corporate bank a new signature specimen, in case cheques I had to sign for my company were rejected. This is the problem with Lyme – how do you convince a doctor that all of these symptoms are not only real, but that they're all related?

I vividly recall shuffling into the bathroom one night, every step hurting and feeling disoriented, lonely, and scared, and saying out loud to my empty apartment, "What is happening to me?" My entire body hurt after sleeping—the longer I lay in one position, the worse the pains. My right hip consistently throbbed for the first hour and a half after I got up.

Hoping to avoid the exodus on the "underground railroad" to the United States that other Lyme victims took, I requested a referral to one of Canada's top infectious disease doctors, who was based at a hospital in Toronto. I was lucky enough to have him agree to see me; however, his acceptance came with the caveat: "I will assess Bob for everything *but* Lyme." At this point, I had the positive IGeneX diagnosis in hand, and I had already cost our medical system thousands of dollars going through a process of elimination of the diseases that Lyme mimics. Nevertheless, one of Canada's supposed infectious disease experts outright refused to consider that I might have Lyme disease. On the other hand, he was clearly willing to spend, and waste, more taxpayer dollars. I won't name and shame him, but in a 2005 interview in a Toronto newspaper article on Lyme disease, he is quoted as saying, "Lyme disease is the most over-diagnosed disease in North America. Even if you did test positive on a Lyme disease test, I would test you again and again and again." I can't even imagine any medical professional speaking this way about any other disease.

The conventional medical system appears to have several problems with Lyme disease. First off, many doctors seem to simply not believe it exists in Canada, and that no bacteria could result in such a disparate, diverse set of symptoms. Compounding that stance is a huge debate within the medical profession over how long to administer antibiotics. Most doctors seem to agree that if Lyme disease is caught early, then an immediate short-term dose of antibiotics will cure it. Doctors who are "Lyme-literate" believe that patients who are still exhibiting symptoms after six weeks of antibiotics haven't been treated long enough. However, the majority of doctors, including the unnamed expert from Toronto, appear to believe that a patient who hasn't recovered after a few weeks of antibiotic treatment is suffering from the aftershocks of the now-cured disease, or from some other unknown reason. For example, many doctors believe that continuing symptoms may be due to an autoimmune response triggered by the initial infection, and therefore continuing antibiotics is not only pointless but potentially harmful. According to this concept, chronic Lyme simply does not exist. Those on either side of the argument can point to numerous studies to support their viewpoint. This results in many physicians being poorly informed or simply scared or unwilling to treat their patients. Caught in this battle are the Lyme patients, forcing them to have to advocate for themselves when they are least able to do so.

One day while I was venting to my daughter Candace about this frustrating battle which I found myself in, she said something profound that really put our health care system into perspective for me: "Dad, you would have been better off to go to a veterinarian." Ontario veterinarians treat dogs for Lyme disease and even vaccinate them against it, while simultaneously the Ontario medical system downplays or outright denies its existence.

Not willing to go back to square one and have to deal with this "expert" doctor who clearly didn't believe in the existence of Lyme disease, I declined the consultation. I had what I thought was a brainstorm: perhaps if I saw a younger doctor, one who had recently graduated, he or she would be savvier and more up to date on Lyme. I booked an appointment with a young doctor only a few years out of medical school and very quickly realized that my brainstorm was wrong. Her only advice, delivered with a smirk on her face, was "If you're spending all that money in the U.S., all I can say is buyer beware." I was getting tired of seeing this smirk from our medical professionals. I responded that if she could spend five minutes in my body, she wouldn't be smirking like she was. At least she had enough shame to blush and look embarrassed at that comment.

Some people have found relief from their Lyme symptoms with the therapeutic use of cannabis, and desperate for any help, I decided to give it a shot. Being highly averse to smoking, and to the smell of cannabis, I acquired some cannabis cookies so that I could ingest the plant in an enjoyable way. Unaware of the potency, I ate an entire cookie as dessert after dinner. Half an hour later I found I was starving, even though I'd just eaten. I went into the bathroom and saw that my pupils were the size of saucers. I suddenly realized why I was starving again: I had the "munchies!" As I walked back to the living room, the floor tilted and I felt like I was on a ship in big seas. In hindsight, one bite would have been a safer bet until I determined the strength of the cookies. Unfortunately, this experience freaked me out sufficiently to curb my curiosity about pot-cookies, but did nothing for my pain.

I found my illness totally consumed my life and left me feeling completely out of control. In addition to my struggles with the medical system, I also had to fight inner battles on multiple fronts: against over-whelming fatigue and exhaustion, against anxiety and non-stop pain, against embarrassing and frustrating cognitive challenges, against the stress and frustration that I couldn't cope with my job, and, finally, against outbursts of raging anger triggered by trifles. Having "brain fog" and unstable emotions certainly didn't help me in dealing with the medical system, or in coping with doctors' smirks and dismissive comments. It was a major challenge to know how to cope with both my physical and emotional reality and, at the same time, a medical system that didn't believe me.

However, learn to cope I did. At this point I would like to digress and acknowledge the one person who has inspired me to persevere: a person just as chronically ill as me, if not more so. In spite of her challenges, she never complains, maintains a positive attitude, and gets on with her life as best as she can. I can't thank enough my inspirational, amazing, loving daughter Candace Osborne Bell, who painted the cover art of this book for me.

Candace lives with Crohn's disease, an autoimmune disease for which the medical community insists there is no cure. The standard treatment for Crohn's, at the level of severity that Candace experiences, is medication to suppress the immune system by targeting specific proteins in the body. The idea behind autoimmune conditions is that the immune system fails to correctly differentiate between self and non-self, and therefore the confused immune system attacks not only foreign substances but also the body's own tissues. It follows, then, that dampening the immune system's ability to function is one way to control symptoms. It should come as no surprise that this approach comes with its own set of risks and side-effects. Beyond the usual complications that can be expected, Candace had additional strange and extreme physical reactions to the drug she was prescribed, and she soon had a whole new set of symptoms about as unpleasant as those of the disease the drug was supposed to control. When she expressed concern to her medical specialist that the drug was causing these new symptoms, she was told that this couldn't be, and that surely this was her disease breaking through, and that she therefore needed *more* of the drug to control these new problems. Having never experienced anything like these new symptoms before, Candace was sure they were side-effects of the drug and elected to wean herself off the medication of her own accord. She tapered off the drug, and all the strange new symptoms went away.

Not one to give up easily, Candace has learned to manage her Crohn's as best she can with diet and lifestyle practices, carefully monitoring practically every bite of food and drop of drink she consumes. One mistake can ruin the rest of the day for her, or in more severe cases, leave her bedridden for days on end. As careful as she is, the cumulative damage caused by the relentless Crohn's continues. It led to her having surgery in 2020 to remove a highly inflamed, scarred section of small bowel.

Candace's health has motivated her to seek further education. Already in possession of an honours Bachelor of Fine Arts degree with a minor in English, she went back to school and became a certified Holistic Nutritionist. She now devotes her limited energy to teaching and helping others. I have learned so much from Candace, not just through her encyclopedic knowledge of nutrition and diet, but most importantly, through how she deals with chronic pain and illness. Candace has found a graceful balance between acceptance and optimism, always striving to improve and do the best she can, while also being gentle and realistic with herself about her needs in a given moment. Rather than fighting herself, she knows that her body is doing its best and has gratitude for all that she is still capable of. Candace, you are my hero and inspiration! I'm still too quick to complain and get into a pity-party, but I'd be a lot worse without my role model to emulate.

I find it intriguing that Canada's provincial and federal governments, and medical community, are reluctant to admit that Lyme can be contracted here, while we suffer the highest rates of MS in the world. The usual explanation for this is that, living in our northern latitudes, we do not get enough Vitamin D from our low sunlight. My counter argument is that there are hundreds of millions of people in Europe living farther north than most Canadians. Europe boasts a deceptively mild climate, thanks to warming caused by the Gulf Stream. As a result, most people don't realize that much of Europe is farther north than southern Canada. The latitude of London, England, is not much south of Thompson, Manitoba (760 kilometres north of Winnipeg), which in some areas had permafrost the last time I was up there. It is well known that Lyme symptoms often mimic those of multiple sclerosis. It makes me wonder how many Canadian MS sufferers might actually be misdiagnosed Lyme victims.

Unfortunately, my experience with the Ontario medical system is not unique, and is apparently still the standard operating procedure that anyone with Lyme disease has to put up with. In December 2018, the *Toronto Star* published an excellent article that chronicled the frustrating experiences of three patients with Lyme disease. The article also quotes my Lyme doctor, Plattsburgh, New York-based Lyme expert Dr. Maureen McShane, as well as the CEO of IGeneX. Sadly, all three people profiled in the article went through experiences similar to mine, including developing mysterious symptoms, difficulty in getting a diagnosis, reluctance or refusal by doctors to treat them, and ultimately being forced to spend tens to hundreds of thousands of dollars on treatment outside of Canada.

Having gone as far I could within my own medical system, I realized I had no choice but to seek expert help outside Canada. I placed myself on

Dr. McShane's waiting list. At that time, she had 1,500 Lyme patients, more than ninety percent of whom were Canadian. My first appointment was in November 2014, during which she diagnosed me with Lyme as well as several co-infections. The ticks don't just pass on the Lyme bacteria; they also generously share other bacteria and parasites, each of which presents its own symptoms as so-called co-infections. My non-medical guess is that the reason every Lyme patient presents with a slightly different or unique smorgasbord of symptoms is the variety of co-infections possible, and the variable ratio of the resulting toxic load.

Dr. McShane reached her diagnosis primarily based on my symptoms, combined with the IGeneX lab results. This diagnosis came thirteen months after my symptoms first appeared, even though I had been aggressively advocating for my health that entire time. As I have already stressed, Lyme is apparently highly curable if caught and treated immediately. Dr. McShane advised me that the odds of recovery are typically eighty to eighty-five percent, but these odds decreased the longer it took to begin treatment following the onset of symptoms. She added that this wasn't always the case; occasionally a patient ill for thirty years would get better faster than someone ill for only two years. My clairvoyant friend had been extremely prescient when she had so adamantly urged me to seek medical advice as soon as possible.

I won't go into a detailed description of Lyme disease and its treatment. I'm a geologist, not a doctor. There are plenty of excellent books and numerous websites that can provide reams of valuable information. Besides, anyone with Lyme disease who is reading this book already knows all of this. Most likely they will have had the same experience as I did and have become self-educated so as to advocate for themselves. On the other hand, I do want to relate my personal experience so that those who are wary of contracting Lyme can know what to look for in terms of symptoms and brace themselves for the inevitable challenges in navigating the medical system.

I will never forget that first trip to upstate New York to see Dr. McShane in November 2014. When I crossed the border, the American customs agent asked me the purpose of my trip. I said I had a doctor's appointment in Plattsburgh, and he immediately replied, "Oh, you must have Lyme!" I subsequently crossed the border for further appointments at two other border crossings, and at each had the same response. What an indictment of our medical system, that so many Canadians have to go out of the country for Lyme treatment that the American border personnel are aware of it.

To give you an idea of how bad I was feeling in late 2014 when I first saw Dr. McShane, I will relate just one example. My son Trevor and I had always thoroughly enjoyed the annual world junior hockey championship, which typically runs from Christmas to early in the new year. It was an opportunity to see future National Hockey League (NHL) all-stars before they became big names; kids playing for their pride in their flag. Cynical Trevor likes to point out that they are also playing for an NHL contract! Toronto co-hosted, along with Montreal, the 2014–2015 championships. Over a year and a half in advance, prior to developing Lyme, I had purchased, at considerable expense, a pair of tickets for every game played in Toronto. In late December 2014, Trevor and I attended the first game in which Canada played. It was all I could do to sit through it, especially since we had a row of young men next to us who were heavily imbibing. Almost constantly one or more were exiting and returning, either on a mission to buy more beer or to visit the washroom. The physical act of standing up was very difficult for me, and they clearly expressed their frustration with how slow I was to stand up and make room for them to pass, to the point where Trevor interceded on my behalf. Following that game, I told Trevor I couldn't handle any more, and, being the wonderful son he is, he did not complain, or at least hid his disappointment well, when I said I planned on selling my remaining tickets. I can't think of a better way of conveying how lousy I felt, that Canada played for the gold medal championship less than a kilometre from my condo, in a game for which I had tickets, and yet I elected not to go.

I hope that gives you an idea of the condition of this patient Dr. McShane met for the first time a month prior. In addition to the cocktail of drugs she prescribed, Dr. McShane also put me on a strict diet, something close to the "paleolithic diet" (which is to imply eating like an ancestral caveman), with no processed food of any kind permitted. Basically, any food in a package, excepting a specific can or a box here or there, was verboten: I was not allowed any sugar, starch, or yeast. I had to avoid all sugar because it feeds the bacteria; therefore, for example, no alcohol, chocolate, salad dressing, mayonnaise, ketchup, mustard, fruit, honey, or maple syrup. The low-starch and yeast-free diet was to prevent any dreadful side effects as a result of taking massive doses of antibiotics. Foods that I could eat would make a shorter list than the forbidden list. Permitted foods included meat, cruciferous vegetables, salad, some whole wheat pasta and brown rice. I could eat tortillas instead of bread, and the occasional yam instead of potatoes. My weight dropped from 196 pounds to 169 pounds in less than two months without doing any exercise. The drastic weight loss only ended when Irina pointed out that I was not eating any carbohydrates at all. I had missed the fact that brown rice and whole wheat pasta were allowed. Once I added them back into my diet my weight stabilized, but it certainly made me think that Weight Watchers has nothing on Dr. McShane's Lyme diet. Maintaining the diet was a lot of work, since I had to map out and plan meals well in advance. Breakfast and lunch essentially consisted of leftovers from dinner.

The first two weeks of drug treatment were mostly anti-fungal and probiotic types of drugs, to prepare my system for the coming onslaught of antibiotics. I then added an anti-malaria pill twice a day, and then slowly ramped up to three different antibiotics. The anti-malaria drug is administered to treat one of the more common co-infections to Lyme, Babesia, a piroplasm (parasite), which Dr. McShane had diagnosed as me having. At one point, I was up to about sixteen antibiotic pills a day (multiple pills of three to five different antibiotics), eighty or so supplements, and over two hundred drops of various herbals and other Lyme-specific remedies. In total, I was taking drugs more than seventeen times a day.

Good thing I've got a cast-iron gut. Other people with Lyme disease I talked with told me their systems couldn't handle the antibiotics. They had to either give up or take them intravenously, which I understand can be dangerous and requires frequent blood monitoring. I had to get bloodwork done once a month just to make sure the heavy-duty load of antibiotics wasn't ruining my kidneys or liver. This was a condition of keeping my doctor; I would be "fired" as her patient if I didn't do so. Canadians are just not as litigious as Americans, so I was not used to dealing with doctors fearing litigation. It would never cross my mind to sue the person trying to help me get better; I knew the risks but thought the potential reward of recovering was well worth it.

Having an American doctor require monthly bloodwork meant I needed my naturopathic doctor to give me the lab requisition form, as no conventional medical doctor would do so. I would then have to pay for the bloodwork, since it had not been ordered by a doctor within our government-funded medical system, and then wait for the naturopath to receive the results and forward them to me. I then forwarded them to Dr. McShane. Such convoluted procedures are difficult and cumbersome at the best of times, let alone when your mind is lost in a shroud of brain fog.

I got my first bloodwork results back on New Year's Eve 2014 and forwarded them immediately to Dr. McShane. She sent me a quick email reply, telling me to "get off the antibiotics, get this kidney detox kit, take it for a week, get another blood test, and then we'll see when you can resume treatment." I was so disappointed, as I thought the treatment was working because I was "herxing." This is slang for a Jarisch-Herxheimer reaction, which means experiencing highly amplified, much worse physical symptoms and pains while on a medical treatment, such as taking large doses of antibiotics. The concept is that when the antibiotics are working well, there is a massive die-off of bacteria. As they die, the bacteria dump their toxins into your bloodstream and overload your body's ability to process and eliminate them.

After ten days of kidney detox, I had another blood test. I failed it as well; my kidneys were still not right. I had to continue on a new regimen of kidney detox before yet another round of retesting, and the third time was the charm, with all systems go to resume treatment. The antibiotics were modified and I restarted treatment. I had an appointment with Dr. McShane every three months; these alternated between being in-person at her office and via telephone consultation. The antibiotics she prescribed were changed both in type, dosage, and frequency from time to time, to fight the various forms the Lyme bacteria can assume. One antibiotic I was on for a while could prove fatal if any alcohol was consumed. The doctor's notes to me included the warning, in block capital letters: DO NOT USE MOUTHWASH. Even though you don't swallow mouthwash, the alcohol in it could cause problems when absorbed through the mouth's surfaces. Irina warned me that this was an extremely strong antibiotic that she only prescribed to dental patients with horrendous infections that had to be staunched quickly, and that I must take the no-drinking warning very seriously.

All this time, fatigue continued to overwhelm me. I "hit the wall" every day at about noon and had to leave my office to go home for a nap. I struggled to juggle work and maintain my drug regimen and dietary restrictions. I had to create a massive spreadsheet to keep track of my medications, and I found that it was almost impossible to work at my office and maintain the medication schedule. I'd get busy in meetings or on the phone, and next thing I knew I'd missed several of the many appointed times per day to take my pills or drops. What follows is an example of my daily schedule.

TIME	DRUG	QUANTITY PILLS	QUANTITY DROPS	COMMENT
Wake-up	Vitamin B6	1		50 mg
	SyCircue	1		dissolve under tongue
	Pekana Big 3		15	drops of each in water
20 MINS Pre-breakfast	BAB-2		6	drops in water
	Wobenzyme	1		
Between first and second bites of breakfast	Nyastin	1		
	Hydroxychloroquine	1		200 mg
	Clarithromycin	2		2 x 250 mg
	Metronidazole	1		250 mg Mon and Tues
	Amoxicillin	3		3 x 500 mg
	Custom formula	4		
	Pancreatic Enzyme	1		
	Malarone	2		
End breakfast	Sacharomyces/HMF Intensive	1		S on M, W, F, HMF on T, T, S, S
10:00 AM	Proteoxyme	2		
	Pekana Big 3		15	drops of each in water
	SyCircue	1		dissolve under tongue
	Boluoke	1		
20 minutes pre-lunch	Wobenzyme	1		
Start lunch	Nourish	3		
	Nyastin	1		
	Omega 3	2		
	Pancreatic Enzyme	1		
	Pekana Big 3		15	drops of each in water
End lunch	Sacharomyces/HMF Intensive	1		S on M, W, F, HMF on T, T, S, S

TIME	DRUG	QUANTITY PILLS	QUANTITY DROPS	COMMENT
03:00 PM	SyCircue	1		dissolve under tongue
	Pekana Big 3		15	drops of each in water
	Boluoke	1		
20 MINS Pre-dinner	BAB-2		6	drops in water
	Wobenzyme	2		
	Proteoxyme	2		
Between first and	Nyastin	1		
second bites of	Hydroxychloroquine	1		200 mg
dinner	Clarithromycin	2		2 x 250 mg
	Metronidazole	1		250 mg Mon and Tues
	Amoxicillin	3		3 x 500 mg
	Malarone	2		
	Pancreatic Enzyme	1		
	Custom formula	4		
End dinner	Sacharomyces/HMF Intensive	1		S on M, W, F, HMF on T, T, S, S
Bedtime	Wobenzyme	4		
	Vitamin B6	1		50 mg
During the night	Activated charcoal	4		
	Microchitasan	2		
	TOTAL	65	72	

In addition to the challenges of working and maintaining the drug regimen, business lunches, dinners, and travel became more and more problematic, given the strict diet I was on. I previously mentioned that one of my Lyme symptoms was emotional instability. I developed a strong social anxiety, including stress at being in noisy crowds and intolerance of noise in general. Conferences, airports, travel, business meetings, and dinners were all essential components of my job. I started to feel that I was not fulfilling my role as CEO and certainly not giving the appropriate time, energy, and effort required. At the same time, I realized that this stress was detrimental to my potential recovery. Ultimately, it became obvious that I could not continue in this manner. I wasn't helping my company or myself. Thanks to the generosity of the chair of the board, Terry, and my wonderfully supportive board of directors, I was put on a six-month sick leave that would allow me to focus solely on recovery. We would re-evaluate my situation afterwards. I commenced this leave in April 2015.

The guy who had been visiting projects in Namibia, Brazil, and Ecuador several times each year had now become a sidelined patient, sitting at home and popping massive doses of drugs. As a geologist, I had always wanted to be taken out by a tiger or anaconda, not by a lowly tick! This was a make-or-break "time out"; if I didn't improve considerably during my six months off, then I'd have to reassess my future.

Early in this book, I mentioned that a common peeve of those living with chronic pain is that well-meaning friends often say, "Oh, but you look so good!" This can make it seem like they believe that it's all in your head, but, of course, they're just trying to make you feel better. I'm sure this is a common feeling among people dealing with a disease that doesn't actually make you look sick; for example, chronic fatigue syndrome or fibromyalgia. I learned to take these comments for the encouragement that they were meant to be as I focused on healing. The days and weeks flew by in a blur of drugs and bloodwork and preparing acceptable meals. Thankfully, I have so many interests and hobbies that I was never bored. After a lifetime of being a workaholic, the enforced free time allowed me to complete a number of projects that I had always wanted to do. I created a database inventory of my stamp collection, working away at it on a pace that I could handle, between daily afternoon naps and adhering to my drug schedule. I spent many hours watching educational DVDs from a company called The Great Courses; as you can imagine they were all science oriented, on subjects such as astronomy, geology, physics, time, and evolution. Highly educational and yet entertaining for a guy like me. One previous passion that I couldn't revive, given that I was living on the 33rd floor of a condo, was watching birds come to my backyard feeders. I had always enjoyed this, especially prior to my divorce, at my last house in Oakville, Ontario, which backed on to a forested ravine. Thanks to this greenspace, my backyard was particularly "birdy." I had loved sitting with my basic point-and-shoot camera, hoping to get decent photos of the various species that dropped by. During my sick leave, it never crossed my mind this interest would soon be revived, and that it would be beneficial to my health.

My six months of sick leave ended in September 2015. Although a bit improved, I was in no shape to fulfill the role I was employed for and knew

I'd have to retire, two years after experiencing my first symptoms. My career ended not with a bang but a whimper. My forced, premature retirement was a double blow—not only was I giving up an exciting career I loved, I was in serious financial jeopardy, given my decision to forego much of my pension when I left Inco, and my recent divorce.

I went through the motions of applying for a disability pension, which was one more exercise in frustration and futility. I was assessed by a doctor working for the insurance company, and when I complained about the blatantly skeptical attitude he had, the company offered a reassessment by a panel of two doctors. They, too, seemed suspicious of my intentions. At one point I asked if they really thought I was pulling a scam. How stupid would I have to be to retire from a well-paying CEO role that I loved, shortly after a divorce, in order to get a tiny disability pension? Rhetorical question, as they denied me anyway. I wonder if anyone has ever received a disability pension for Lyme disease in Canada; based on my experience, I doubt it.

Dealing with the insurance company doctors wasn't the end of challenges that were especially difficult to handle in my condition. My transition into retirement was not without further drama.

Following my divorce in 2012, I had moved from our family home in Oakville to a condo I leased in downtown Toronto. Since my work required me to travel constantly, I didn't want to own a house while living on my own. It would be sitting empty for weeks on end, with telltale signs for burglars such as an uncut lawn, driveway full of snow, and mail or flyers piling up. The condo was situated only a kilometre, about a ten-minute walk, from my office. It was very expensive as it was located right on Lake Ontario, and, being on the 33rd floor, had a stunning view across the Toronto Islands and lake. On cold, clear winter days I could see the mist rising from Niagara Falls, located roughly sixty-five kilometres across Lake Ontario. Now that I was forced into premature retirement, there was no reason to be living in downtown Toronto close to my office, to say nothing of my sudden inability to afford it.

Shortly after moving to Toronto, I had been lucky to meet Irina, who was also a tenant in my condo building. We began dating and had a wonderful time together, with lots of dinners out and weekends away. When I got sick, Irina never hesitated: she would stick with me. While undertaking her dentistry degree, she had taken a number of general medicine courses. So she was a great sounding board when I had questions or needed to vent my frustrations. She was able to give me excellent advice, particularly on the antibiotics I was being prescribed by my Lyme doctor, as she had prescribed some of them to her own patients. As I mentioned earlier, when I was at my "Lymiest," we'd go for a walk of maybe 200 metres, Irina half-carrying me and supporting me, and, if we had to climb a hill, literally pushing me from behind to propel me up it.

Fully aware that I'd most likely have to retire at the end of my sick leave, I decided to look for a new home to share with Irina. Based on financial considerations, I knew I had to move outside of the Greater Toronto Area (the "GTA"), and yet not too far for Irina to commute to her dental practice, or too far for me to see my kids, who both live in Toronto. We sat with a map of southern Ontario and placed circles of varying diameters on it, and then selected a few communities that were of potential interest. After a few drives and viewing several homes, we narrowed the search to west of the GTA. I had always loved the Ancaster and Dundas area, just outside of Hamilton, located at the western end of Lake Ontario about eighty kilometres from downtown Toronto. The landscape is beautiful, with its lush primary Carolinian forest and dramatic topography formed by the Niagara Escarpment. I took Irina for a drive one weekend, and as we drove down into the Dundas Valley, she exclaimed, "Bobby, you found me Vancouver Island." When Irina immigrated from Ukraine to Canada, and prior to taking a two-year qualifying course at the University of Toronto's dental school, she had lived in Vancouver for a while. She had missed it, and its milder climate, since heading east to Toronto.

While driving on a road through gorgeous forest, we came upon a house for sale. Given its location, we knew it would be in the multimillion-dollar range, and therefore out of our league, but we decided we should talk to the listing agent. We took down her name and phone number from the sale sign, and I called her the next day. I asked her if there were any townhouse complexes located in a similar forest setting.

Thanks to a few moves I had made on my own, along with numerous corporate relocations over the course of my career, I had previously bought and sold a total of nine houses, but never a townhouse. I decided a condominium townhouse was best for me, in case my health continued to deteriorate. I worried that I wouldn't be able to do any maintenance. With the townhouse, lawn cutting, snow shoveling, and other external maintenance were covered in the monthly condo fee.

The agent explained that townhouse complexes backing onto forest or conservation area were few and far between and highly in demand, given the number of baby boomers who were starting to retire and looking to downsize. We visited a couple of units of interest that had just come on the market the day before, and both already had offers on them before we could even get in the door. We realized that this wasn't going to be easy.

The agent told us of another unit in a forest setting that she knew was for sale and was located only four hundred metres from the old village of Ancaster. On August 18, 2015, we were thrilled to make an offer and have it accepted, with closing slated for September 30. We both gave notice to the owners of our respective apartments that we planned to terminate our leases.

My friend Geoff is a fantastic carpenter and home builder. I wanted his ideas on possible renovations and upgrades prior to moving in. In mid-September, about two weeks prior to closing, I arranged with the vendor and the real estate agent to gain access to the house and lined up Geoff to meet us there.

At the house, I noticed a large poster in the front window but didn't look closely at it. The real estate agent had the key from the vendor, but it wouldn't work in the lock. We then noticed a large pile of iron filings on the front step under the door. At this point I took a serious look at the poster and saw that it was an eviction notice to have all contents removed by a certain date. Totally confused, the agent called the vendor, who claimed to be unaware of what might have transpired. We sat in a gazebo in the lovely communal gardens across from the unit, waiting for him to show up. After seeing the notice and realizing that the lock had been drilled out and changed, he admitted that his business was on the verge of bankruptcy. He had placed several mortgages and liens on the house to borrow money to prop up his business. The bank had clearly foreclosed on him and seized the house. As my lawyer said to me, "Bob, I've had lots of real estate purchases fall through because the purchaser could not secure financing. Never in thirty years have I seen a deal not close because the vendor lost title."

The retirement home I'd purchased was not meant to be. By coincidence, the bank that seized the house was the same bank with which I had already secured a mortgage to make the purchase. Try as I might, they would not put me in the front of the line to buy it, saying there was a strict firewall between divisions within the bank.

Irina and I both scrambled to reverse our notices to move out. The fellow I was leasing from would extend my lease only if I would commit to a minimum of six months. Legally, I could have fought him, as under Ontario law, after one year you can renew on a monthly basis. Irina had no trouble doing exactly that. There was no way I was going to commit to six months, as at that point I was still naively hoping that I could purchase the house once the bank listed it. We decided I'd move into Irina's, which was a smaller apartment than mine. Thus began my retirement at the age of 58; a rather ignoble start after a thirty-five-year career.

I was despairing over losing this townhouse that was in such a unique setting, secluded in a forest, yet only a few minutes' walk to most amenities. A number of well-meaning friends and family tried to console me by stating that we'd lost the house for a reason, that it wasn't meant to be, and that, furthermore, it meant that something even better might come along. *Bah humbug* was all I could think. We'd been told there was very little turnover in the complex, and huge competition to get in. Long story short, my real estate agent caught wind that another unit in the same complex, one with a more secluded backyard, was going to be sold. She arranged for us to see it before it was publicly listed. Within seconds of walking in and having a quick glance about, seeing the wall of green trees and bushes outside the large living room windows, we locked eyes and could instantly read each other's minds. This was it. Although Irina probably wasn't envisioning bird feeders, like I was!

As mentioned earlier, we had previously visited two homes that were sold within a day of listing. This made negotiating simple; we knew that if we were going to get this place, the best (and only) way to secure it was to simply accept the vendor's selling price. Haggling would only leave us open to being outbid by others. Although quite a bit more expensive than the unit we had lost, I had previously secured financing to mortgage it and was confident that there would be no issue getting a larger mortgage. I took a gamble and accepted his selling price, unconditionally. To make it conditional on financing meant another buyer could pre-empt us by making an unconditional offer. And so, just like that, on a handshake we had the house, with sixty days' closing, meaning we could move in on December 10. My well-meaning friends' predictions had come true: we lost the first unit for a reason. The moral of the story? Maybe some things are meant to be ... and maybe my contracting Lyme disease was meant to be in order for me to become a passionate birder.

As soon as we moved in, my retirement could officially begin.

5. ADJUSTING TO RETIREMENT

Now that I was truly retired, I consulted with Dr. McShane, and we agreed that I would cease treatment. I had been highly incentivized to get better, as I did not want to retire, mainly because I loved what I did, but just as important, I wasn't in a financial position to retire. With those incentives gone, I really didn't want to continue to subject my body to such massive doses of antibiotics, and quite honestly, I couldn't afford the continued cost. I would concede that Lyme had won the first round, knocking me out of work, but I refused to let it win any more rounds. I would try to learn to live with chronic pain and fatigue and accept that as my new permanent condition. One downside of going off the treatment was that my weight very quickly returned to about 195 pounds.

The problem with condos is that they come with rules. Before buying the first unit that we ultimately lost, I had my lawyer confirm there was no stipulation against bird feeders. Thankfully it was still quite warm in December 2015 when we moved in, so one of the first things I did was to buy a new bird-feeding station and set it up before the ground was frozen.

The original occupants of our unit had had a say in the layout and design. The lady had some mobility issues, so they designed it such that their master bedroom was on the ground level, with large windows looking out to a very secluded backyard with several large maple trees and three spruce trees. These trees provided not only a level of privacy unheard of for a townhouse, but a fantastic staging area for birds to hide in and feel secure as they visited my feeders. Irina agreed that this master bedroom would be an ideal office for my very large desk and bookshelves. Hence, as I write this, I'm sitting at my desk looking straight out to dozens of birds congregating at our feeders and in the surrounding trees.

The forest in which our townhouse complex is located connects indirectly to the 1,200-hectare Dundas Valley Conservation Area. The Dundas Valley is what geologists call a re-entrant valley. On a map it is C-shaped, with the C formed by the Niagara Escarpment. Ancaster is located on top of the escarpment at the bottom of the C, and the valley is in the middle of the C. The result of glaciation and the unique geology which creates the escarpment, the valley hosts meadows and Carolinian forest—one of the last remnants of it preserved in southern Ontario. The lush forest contains numerous species of trees rare or unheard of in the rest of Canada, such as American sycamore, tulip-tree, sassafras, cucumber magnolia, paw-paw, and flowering dogwood, as well as more common white pines, hemlock, maples and oaks. The combination of unique topography, a relatively warmer climate than most of Ontario, mixed deciduous-coniferous forest, along with secondary successional growth over old orchards and previously cleared farmland, results in a variety of habitats that attract and sustain numerous bird species. In addition, the topography leads to the city of Hamilton's claim to be the "Waterfall Capital of the World," with about 130 waterfalls within the city limits. All of this running water and numerous creeks are also key to attracting and sustaining a huge variety of bird species.

Migrating birds try to minimize the amount of open water they have to fly across, for obvious safety reasons. I created the following image using Google Earth to depict the routing of northbound birds during spring migration. As you can see, Lake Erie has a couple of short cuts across it, which explains why Long Point and Point Pelee are excellent, world-famous locations for birding during migration. Lake Ontario does not have similar shortcuts. However, the Niagara Peninsula, extending between the southwestern shore of Lake Ontario and the northeastern shore of Lake Erie, offers a great corridor for migrating birds; it is more an isthmus than a peninsula, serving as a land link that allows birds to avoid having to fly across Lake Ontario. The result is that many northbound migrating birds in spring that hit Lake Ontario or the eastern end of Lake Erie will turn to detour and funnel across the Niagara Peninsula, making for great birding. Raptors such as hawks and eagles in particular utilize the peninsula, as they can ride the thermal air currents that rise up off Lake Ontario over the Niagara Escarpment, thus getting a bit of a free ride. The same principle applies to southbound birds during fall migration; just imagine the arrow directions reversed. Our Ancaster home is located at the western end of Lake Ontario.

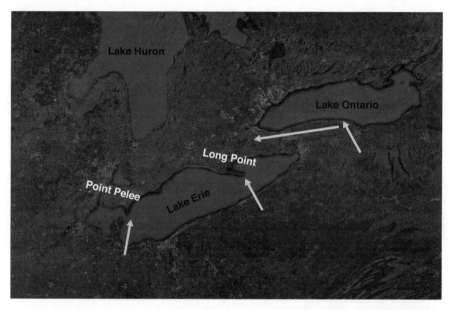

The Niagara Peninsula allows birds to avoid crossing the lakes
(Created using Google Earth)

As a result of this favorable location for birds, during our first winter in our new home I was delighted by the numerous species that came to my feeders, including one new to me, the Carolina Wren. Like its namesake forest, the wren is here on the northern limit of its range. Being a scientist and always eager to learn, I decided to write a book for myself on the birds I could expect in our area. My book was simply a compilation of information from numerous sources that I pulled together and assembled, customized to the birds of Ancaster and surrounding areas. As a student, I always found the best way to learn was to write out notes, so by writing the book I gained considerable knowledge without leaving the comfort of my home.

As I wrote and researched, I was watching my feeders and enjoying every minute of it. I was finding that my body was not screaming at me while I was either learning about birds or watching them, or if it was, I wasn't aware of it. I was discovering something that was to me more powerful than antibiotics: a new "treatment plan," one self-administered and with no detrimental side effects. This treatment would involve a return to nature and to the great outdoors. It was like my career as a geologist, but rather than figuring out what a certain rock or mineral was, I was learning various bird species, their songs, and habits. My dad would have been proud that the love of nature and science he had instilled in me was now beneficial to my well-being. This new hobby is obviously not a cure for Lyme, but rather a coping mechanism to deal with chronic illness and pain. Birding is—or at least has been for me—a way of keeping life full of mystery and excitement, and diverting my mind from my aching body.

Of the thirty-six units in our townhouse complex, only one or two others had feeders out. I started to hear complaints about woodpeckers doing damage to the stucco siding of a few units. There were a few "joking" comments that the problems didn't start until I moved in and put up my feeders. As I already mentioned, the downside to condo living is that there are rules. Next thing I knew, there was a debate and consideration was given to banning birdfeeders. This was going to be on the agenda of the Annual General Meeting (AGM). I had thought that with retirement I was done with worrying about potential dramas at AGMs, such as irate shareholders.

Scrambling to prepare for the meeting, I found a research paper from the Cornell Lab of Ornithology that showed that, though the results were not definitive, there was no significant correlation between woodpecker attacks and the presence of bird feeders, and in fact, if anything, there was a slightly lesser chance of a woodpecker attack if feeders are present. If you're a woodpecker, why beat your head against a house if there is suet or other free food put out for you? I also sought and received a great supporting email from an ornithologist at Bird Studies Canada (now Birds Canada). At the AGM I gave an impassioned defence of birds, telling my neighbours that the birds aren't in our backyards, we are in theirs, so if you don't like nature, you shouldn't be living in a forest. After the meeting I put together and distributed to the other thirty-five condo owners a PDF file with photos of my backyard beauties, including a Baltimore Oriole, Rose-breasted Grosbeak, Indigo Bunting, Carolina Wren, Northern Cardinal, and Blue Jay. Many had no idea they were living among so many beautiful birds, and became more interested in them as a result. Not only did I win the day, I was also asked to give a presentation for the residents of our community, which was hosted at the Ancaster library in September 2016. This led to a number of requests from other library branches in the region to give talks on "Backyard Birding and Beyond." My talks even got promoted in a local newspaper: *Get an introduction to birding in the Hamilton area. Learn about the different types of local birds and where you can spot them yourself. See photos of an array of birds spotted in 2016 by birding enthusiast Bob Bell from the Hamilton Naturalists' Club. Presented By: Bob Bell, Hamilton Naturalists' Club.* I will touch on the Hamilton Naturalists' Club and its positive influence on me in the next chapter.

I have had two heartwarming experiences as a result of giving these library talks. The first came after a presentation I gave in May 2017. I would always give my email address at the end of my talk and invite audience members to contact me if they had any questions. The next day, I received the following email from a woman who had attended:

> *Thank you for your presentation yesterday. I learned a great deal and thoroughly enjoyed your photos. Your photos had a way of not only showing the beauty of the bird but also so much of its unique personality. I also liked that you provided a list of areas for birdwatching.*
>
> *For years now, I have so wanted to see an Eastern Bluebird and have yet to see one in my life. If you could please let me know where I might go to see one. I have found out about the nature hikes with Hamilton Nature but the issue is that I am not able to go on any of their 2-hour hikes-- about 45 minutes would be my limit right now. I would greatly appreciate if you knew of any other hikes or options for me to see a bluebird. I look forward to hearing from you.*

I happened to know of a nearby location where there was a bluebird nesting box just inside a farm field fence. One could drive right to it and not even have to get out of the car to see both the male and female catching insects to feed their young. I sent detailed directions and a week later got this response:

> *I saw my first bluebird this morning!! I followed your directions and had no problem finding the birdhouses. When I arrived, I saw a bluebird*

*immediately right at the birdhouse and then it quickly flew away. I could
see the beautiful blue as it flew away to the trees of the farm across the
road. It was extremely windy so decided to turn my car around and
watch from my car directly across. I arrived at 9:45 a.m. and watched
for 1/2 hour. During that time, the bluebirds came back about three times.
Sometimes they would sit on top of the post or on the wire fence as well.
It was pure joy to experience this.*

*I cannot thank you enough for your support and encouragement.
When I was leaving there, I thought ... wait until I tell Bob!*

*How long do you think these bluebirds will be there for? Do they
all leave once the young birds are ready to fly? I forgot my binoculars and
took a photo only at a distance. I couldn't even come close to the quality
of your photos.*

*Before this morning, as you know, I had never seen a real bluebird.
Now I have an experience I will always remember. Thank you again.*

Her sheer joy and exhilaration at seeing a bluebird came through
loud and clear. I was very touched reading this; to think that I, a neophyte
birder, had managed to make someone so happy, and to hear the passion
and appreciation in her words. This hooked me even more on birding, and
on sharing my birding experiences with others.

The second experience, which occurred in early 2020, also involved,
coincidentally, bluebirds. I had stopped at a local site where there was a
small flock of overwintering bluebirds. A younger couple with their son,
about eleven years old at the time, came along and stood next to me as we
scanned the field looking for them. The young lad held a field notebook
and had binoculars strung around his neck. He announced that he could
hear them chattering as they flew overhead; looking up, I saw that he was
correct and was instantly impressed with his knowledge and observational
skills. As he recorded the sighting in his notebook, his father looked at me
and said "We're here because of you." Seeing the puzzled look on my face,
he went on to explain that they had attended one of my library talks, and
upon leaving the son announced that he wanted to be an ornithologist and
obtain a degree from Cornell University! Apparently, my talk really inspired

and motivated him to expand the interest he obviously already had, to not only become a passionate birder but perhaps make a career of it. Since then, I've seen him make a number of posts to our naturalists' club's email hotline, advising members of some noteworthy sighting. He is already living his dream, having been awarded the top young birder trophy for 2019 in the Hamilton Naturalists' Club, and now authors a birding blog. To learn that I had played a small role in inspiring a member of the next generation to get passionate about birding brought tears to my eyes!

My symptoms seem to have a bit of a seasonal cyclicity to them. Apparently, it is not uncommon for Lyme patients to feel better in the spring and summer and then worse again in the fall and winter. In the fall of 2016, after being off treatment for about eight months, I found myself spiralling down again, so in November I returned to Plattsburgh, New York, to see Dr. McShane. She put me on a new regimen of antibiotics, including Rifampin, which is used for tuberculosis, leprosy, and Lyme. It was much easier to maintain the drug protocol, being at home and retired, though once again I lost a lot of weight on the restricted diet. I probably wasn't quite as religious about it as I was during the first round, and my weight only dropped to about 180 from 195 pounds.

By August 2017, I was feeling a bit better, and Dr. McShane felt that she had done as much as she could for me. When she asked me to put a number on my improvement from my first consultation with her, I estimated that I was sixty percent better. I was a long way from the guy who needed a cane to walk and couldn't count out $1.75 in change, but I was still living with constant muscle and joint pain, shortage of breath, rubbery legs, awful neuropathy, debilitating fatigue, and very erratic emotions. Once again, I was tired of being chained to a tight drug schedule and living on a limited diet, and I was ready to enjoy the occasional glass of red wine (or three!). Dr. McShane recommended that I continue taking my prescriptions and supplements until they ran out, but she wasn't going to prescribe any more. I had an emotional "breakup" with my Lyme doctor, and her parting words of comfort were, "Don't worry, I'm always here for you if you ever need me."

When I came off the strict diet, I made a better effort to not have my weight balloon back to 195. I began a daily workout with light weights and a stability ball, and rode my stationary bike for up to thirty minutes a day. Bread seemed to be the biggest culprit in weight gain, so I continued to eat tortillas instead, with the occasional "cheating" to satisfy my love of toast and bread. These efforts seem to have paid off, and I'm now at a stable 185 pounds. Dr. McShane had suggested that I try taking injections of Vitamin B12 to help my neuropathy. Irina had the lovely task of giving me a shot in the butt every other day for a couple of months. It didn't help.

However, typical of Lyme, I cycled down again. At this point, medical cannabis was legal in Canada. My previous cookie experience had not gone well. However, there seemed to be more than just anecdotal evidence that cannabis helped with pain management, so I requested and got a referral to a clinic that dispensed it. The expert at the clinic recommended that I vape it rather than smoke it, especially after I told her I found smoking disgusting and couldn't stand the smell of cannabis. I bought the equipment and an ounce of medical-grade cannabis (okay, that's a street term; I bought 30 grams), and proceeded to try it. It did nothing for me; it did not touch my pain at all. Shortly after that experiment, I met a friend of my younger sister who was in the business of selling CBD oil (Cannabidiol). CBD is an extract from the cannabis plant, and unlike the compound delta-9 tetrahydrocannabinol (commonly referred to as THC), it is not psychoactive. This means that CBD does not change a person's state of mind when they use it, but it supposedly has health benefits. Again, it did nothing for me. It seemed that my chronic pain, neuropathy, and fatigue were just going to be my new normal, and I'd have to learn to live with them.

The entire time I was going through these treatments to deal with my symptoms, I did as many birding related activities as possible. These included taking online courses, a couple of single-day in-class courses, backyard birding, and hikes and walks with my camera. I was continuously reminded that the one thing that took my mind off my pain was birding.

6. WHY BIRDING?

Many birders refer to their "spark bird," the first bird that really captured their attention and intrigued them so much that they eventually ended up being hooked. I suppose, if pushed, I'd have to say it was seeing my first ever Carolina Wren in the backyard, which led to my researching and writing the book on the birds of the Hamilton area that I mentioned earlier. However, my conversion to being a birder was not really triggered by that wren or any one particular bird; it was a Hamilton Naturalists' Club birding field trip that really solidified an inchoate interest I'd always had. I've previously described the enjoyment and peace of mind that watching my bird feeders and researching birds gave me. The half day field trip took me to a whole different level. I was in the outdoors, enjoying nature with a group of like-minded individuals, not unlike being on a geology field trip to visit a mineral prospect. I was seeing new bird species for the first time. I met Barry Coombs and Peter Thoem, and new friendships were established. I got tips on cameras and binoculars. While all this was occurring, I was unaware of my aching body; instead, I was really enjoying myself.

As a result of that trip, I subsequently bought a camera that had been recommended to me. This led me to undertake more and more walks of greater and greater length, hoping to see and photograph as many birds as possible. I bought a Fitbit to keep track of my excursions and was pleasantly shocked to find that the guy who previously could only walk a few hundred metres with the aid of a cane was routinely walking up to five or more kilometres a day. The Fitbit data proved I was physically improving without even realizing it. As long as the ground was relatively flat, I could plod along happily, listening to and looking for whatever birds I might encounter. It is not that my Lyme symptoms were gone; but they *did* seemingly disappear while my focus was redirected on birds. All my senses were heightened, in a good way—the thrill and satisfaction of stalking and sneaking up on a bird to get a better look at it and to photograph it; the sound of birds singing and the wind whispering in the pines and rustling the leaves; and the feel of fresh air and warm sunshine bathing my face. I knew that these feelings and emotions were mitigating the usual painful sensations that Lyme gave me, and I knew I'd found a hobby I'd happily spend the rest of my life engaged in.

7. BACKYARD BIRDING FOR BEGINNERS

Even if you've never paid attention to a bird in your life, I bet they enter your vocabulary regularly. Here is just a handful of some of my favourite bird-related expressions; for a longer list of all the bird-related idioms and expressions I could think of, see Appendix A at the back of the book.

- The early bird catches the worm
- What's good for the goose is good for the gander
- Don't count your chickens before they hatch
- Birds of a feather flock together
- Like water off a duck's back

Even if you are unaware of it, birds are in your life, whether you like them or not!

At the risk of repeating myself, seeing birds can be very uplifting for your mood, your spirit, your soul, and your body. Once called *birdwatching*, the modern term for this activity is simply *birding*. It sounds much more active and "cooler" than the passive *birdwatching*, which frequently carries a nerd connotation. Birding does not have to be an expensive hobby or require a lot of energy, and it can mean different things to different people. You don't have to go on long, extensive hikes through challenging terrain. If one's health does not permit getting out and walking trails or actively birding, great pleasure can be had in the comfort of your own living room, watching backyard feeders—presuming you live in a house and not an apartment. You can easily entice a few birds to your yard; all it takes is a feeder or two, along with a few trees or shrubs to provide a hiding spot for birds to either sneak up to the feeders or to seek refuge when startled. Considering that at any given time there are between 200 billion and 400 billion individual birds in the world, equating to roughly thirty to sixty birds per human on the planet, surely a few will bless your yard with their appearance.

According to Birds Canada, twenty-five percent of Canadian households have bird feeders or bird houses in their yards. Not surprisingly, the same percentage of Canadians spend a lot of money on bird seed or birding products, averaging $1,000 per year.

Although just a single feeder will do, you will find that different species of birds have different feeding habits and food preferences, so if you want to attract a variety of birds, you will really need a variety of feeder types.

My recommendation is to invest in a feeding station, as shown in the following photo. Modern systems allow for multiple feeders of various styles to be hung from, or attached to, the same central pole. This way you can vary the types of feeders and feed you are putting out, depending on the season or what species of birds you are hoping to attract. I am constantly switching mine up, and will show in detail a few other types of feeders not seen in the setup in the photo. One key element is to have a funnel-like obstacle called a baffle on the main upright pole. This prevents squirrels and racoons from shinnying up the pole and cleaning out the feeders (and your wallet!). As long as the pole is placed a minimum of ten feet from the nearest branches, the squirrels generally can't launch themselves through the air and land on it, either. Another useful "appendage" to attach is a long rod, which I've labeled as "staging area." It is easier to see in the following close-up photos, showing that birds will sit on it while waiting their turn to get at a feeder.

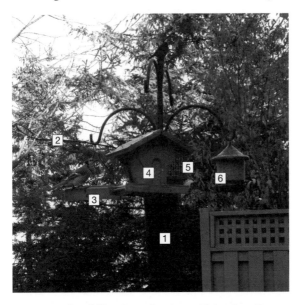

NOT A 'BIRD FEEDER', IT'S A 'FEEDING STATION'

1. Baffle
2. Staging area
3. Platform feeder
4. House feeder
5. Suet feeder
6. Clingers-only feeder

In the following photo, a Chipping Sparrow sits on the staging area arm, looking to see if the coast is clear for his turn.

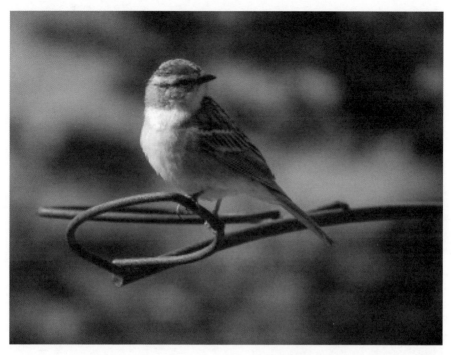

Chipping Sparrow on staging area arm

Much to my shock and delight, in the spring of 2020 a Scarlet Tanager blessed us with a one-day appearance. He had clearly migrated overnight and was in need of refuelling; he spent all day gorging at the feeders.

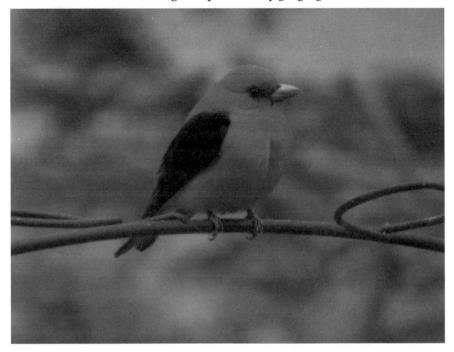

Scarlet Tanager, my best feeder bird ever

Birds will also utilize the top rungs of the feeder station to perch before going to the actual feeder. In this case a Rose-breasted Grosbeak is checking out what is on the menu.

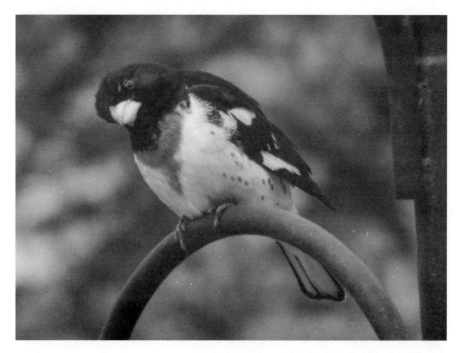

Rose-breasted Grosbeak checking out the menu

Although some bird species are "generalists" in both their diet and feeding style, many are either specialists or have strong preferences. You can find specific feeders for each choice. Some birds are platform feeders, some are ground feeders, and some like to cling, even upside down. I feed birds all year round, whereas many only put their feeders out in the winter, when food is tougher for the birds to come by naturally. Sunflower seeds are probably the most popular item for both the birds and the folks that buy seed. I personally don't like them, as the empty shells make a mess and kill the grass under the feeder. I buy "no mess" chipped sunflower seeds.

I occasionally put out peanut trays, but since peanuts are favoured by many birds, I put the small "rooftop" fairly tight above it, so that nuthatches and wrens can access it, but larger "pig birds" cannot. In the next photo, a cute little Carolina Wren is as snug as a bug sitting in the peanut tray, safe from harassment from larger birds.

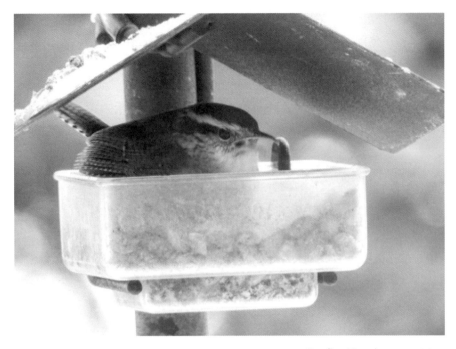

Carolina Wren in a peanut tray

I apologize to pigs; I don't mean to disparage them. My scientific classification of pig birds includes European Starlings, Red-winged Blackbirds, Common Grackles, and Brown-headed Cowbirds. These birds tend to arrive in small to large flocks and, if given their way, would clean everything out in short order. Since most of these species would prefer platforms, I have stopped using an unprotected platform feeder, as seen with a Blue Jay on it in the photo of my feeding station. Instead, I use a "dinner bell" tray feeder with an adjustable dome-like covering, which serves two purposes: one is that it keeps the seed dry in the rain (which is important so that your seed doesn't get moldy), and two, you can adjust the height such that Northern Cardinals, Rose-breasted Grosbeaks, and smaller birds can find their way in, but the larger pig birds cannot. I should add that, like any good parent, I love my children equally, and likewise, I do care about the so-called pig birds. They are still able to get seed off the ground. In the following photo two male Purple Finch are enjoying this feeder.

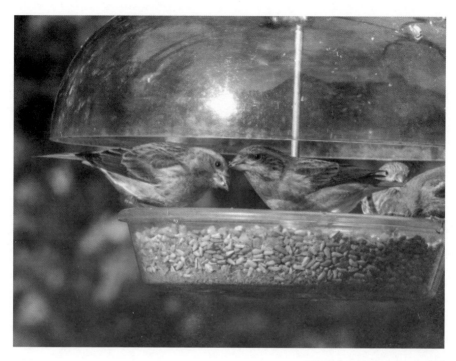

Dinner is served under the bell

Having no open platform feeders really reduces the presence of the pig birds, as well as two other birds that I didn't mention in my pig bird list—Mourning Doves and Rock Pigeons. The latter two are the ultimate pig birds but are too large to land on the feeders I utilize, whereas when I had open platform feeders, they monopolized the feeding station. A favorite tactic of both was to get on an open platform and knock all the seed off, and then contentedly graze away on the ground.

The smaller hanging feeder in the next photo is meant for "clingers" only—Black-capped Chickadees, nuthatches, and some finches. The three birds on it are Pine Siskins, a type of small finch. I've watched Northern Cardinals and Blue Jays successfully get seeds from it, but I'm sure they burn more calories than they consume by frantically flapping to hang on long enough for a morsel.

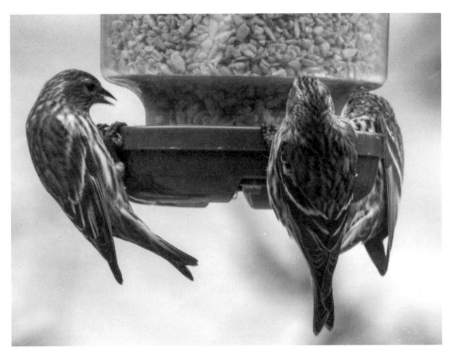

Pine Siskins on a clingers-only feeder

I find that a seed cylinder is a favorite of almost everyone. They are large enough that occasionally two birds can dine together. In the first of the following photos, a Yellow-bellied Sapsucker shares the seed cylinder with a Red-breasted Nuthatch, who is striking a classic upside-down pose, characteristic of this species. The second photo shows a unique opportunity I had to see the size difference between a Downy Woodpecker on the left and the larger Hairy Woodpecker on the right (both females). Unfortunately, at times I've had to temporarily take down my seed cylinders if the pig birds learn how to cling on; after a few days' absence they typically give up and move on, and I can put the cylinders back out.

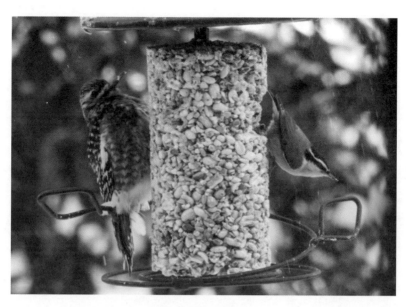

Yellow-bellied Sapsucker and Red-breasted Nuthatch sharing the seed cylinder

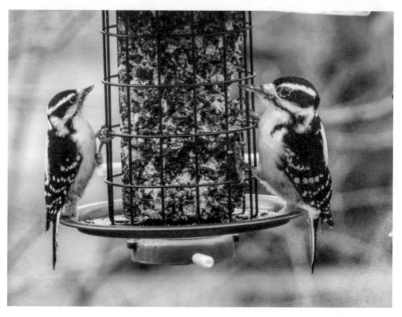

Downy Woodpecker on the left and Hairy Woodpecker on the right

A Nyjer tube feeder is wonderful for finches, particularly American Goldfinches and Pine Siskins in the winter. The next photo, taken in March 2017, shows three scruffy looking American Goldfinch in the midst of moulting into their spring breeding plumage.

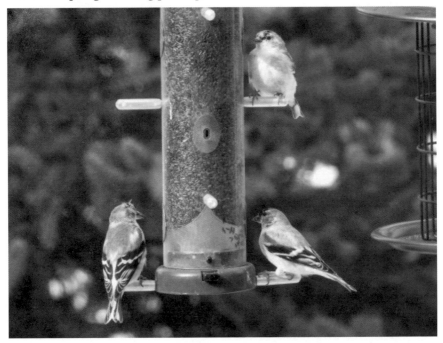

Moulting American Goldfinches enjoying the nyjer feeder

In winters when their food source is poor, there might be an "irruption" of winter finches. This means that birds move further south, out of their normal range in northern boreal forests, in search of food. A Canadian expert has put out a much anticipated annual "finch report" in which he forecasts the likelihood of seeing such birds in the winter based on the abundance of natural foods such as pine cones and birch seeds in their normal range. In the summer of 2020, after twenty-one years, he announced his retirement from this endeavour, disappointing the North American birding community. Fortunately he has passed the reins to another expert who has been working with him, so this invaluable information will continue to be provided. The so-called winter finches which periodically irrupt includes Pine Siskins,

Common Redpolls, Evening Grosbeaks, Pine Grosbeaks, Red Crossbills, and White-winged Crossbills. Red-breasted Nuthatches can also get pushed further south during a big irruption winter. The winter of 2020-2021 was an epic irruption year, with huge numbers of these winter finches showing up well into the central to southern United States. I never dreamed I'd have Evening Grosbeaks and Common Redpolls at my feeders in Ancaster. Normally, by which I mean in pre-pandemic times, I'd make an annual winter trip to Algonquin Park to see these beautiful birds. This winter I just sat at my desk and watched up to forty Common Redpolls out my window, such as this gorgeous fellow.

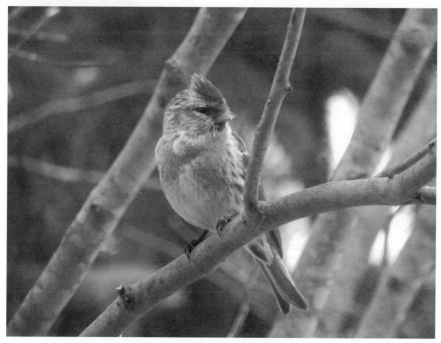

Common Redpoll in southern Ontario during the great irruption of winter 2020-2021

As an aside, the same irruption concept applies to owls that normally inhabit the Arctic or boreal forests, such as Snowy Owls and Great Gray Owls. In a big irruption year, Snowy Owls are frequently found along the shores of all the Great Lakes, and even as far south as Florida. The current understanding of the reason for a Snowy Owl irruption is actually counterintuitive and opposite the reason for a finch irruption. In the Arctic tundra, the main food source for Snowy Owls is lemmings. The lemming population is cyclical over a number of years; when it is high, the Snowy Owls will have greater reproductive success, leading to a higher Snowy Owl population. A higher density of owls means greater competition for food, leading to owls ranging further afield for food. They head south because they've had so much food during the breeding season.

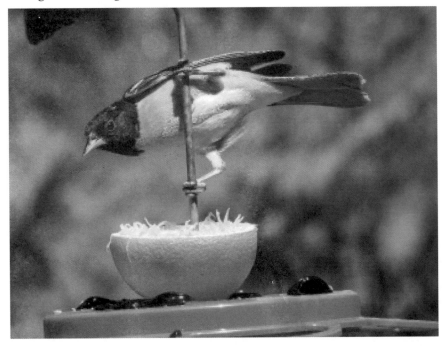

Baltimore Oriole checks out the orange and grape jelly

In the summer, I put out the oriole feeder a few days before I expect them to return from their winter vacation. In addition to oranges, Baltimore Orioles absolutely love grape jelly as you will see in the above photo. I've read articles suggesting this might not be the healthiest for them, but perhaps they are like us humans, who love our sugar-rich snacks in spite of the health risks. The nice thing about the oriole feeder is there is no competition for the Baltimore Orioles; the only other birds I've seen touch the jelly or orange are Ruby-throated Hummingbirds and, bizarrely, a Gray Catbird. Conversely,

I've seen Baltimore Orioles go to my hummingbird feeder. Although it's important to keep all your feeders clean, I think in particular you want to freshen your sugar water for the hummingbirds frequently, if not daily during really warm weather.

Suet feeders are great for woodpeckers, but I find a number of other species, such as Carolina Wrens, will also eat the suet. I particularly like the double suet feeder with the long extended "paddle" at the bottom, which provides a surface for larger woodpeckers to brace their tails against. In the next photo, a Yellow-bellied Sapsucker takes advantage of this feeder.

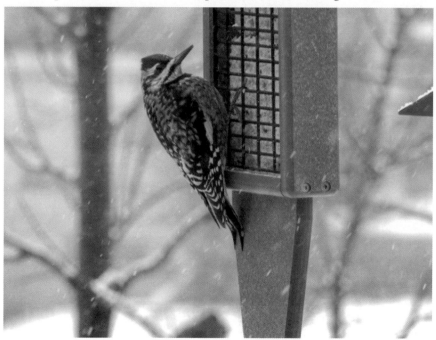

Double suet feeders are great for larger woodpeckers

I only put out suet feeders in the winter, as in the summer suet melts into messy, rancid goo. I also occasionally put out an "upside-down" suet feeder, so that the nimble and dexterous woodpeckers can eat in peace without worrying about raptors catching them or other birds annoying them. A Red-bellied Woodpecker demonstrates this in the following photo.

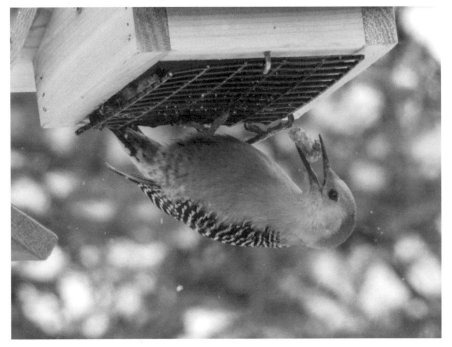

Peace and quiet at the upside-down suet feeder

If you want to entice birds into your backyard, fresh water is almost as important as feeders. My bird bath gets visited by everyone – virtually every species of bird in the yard, as well as the chipmunks and squirrels. Even better would be to have some sort of running water feature, thus ensuring the water is always fresh and clean. The following photo is of a Common Grackle at my birdbath. He's so beautiful, even though he looks rather cranky, that I almost feel guilty referring to him as a pig bird.

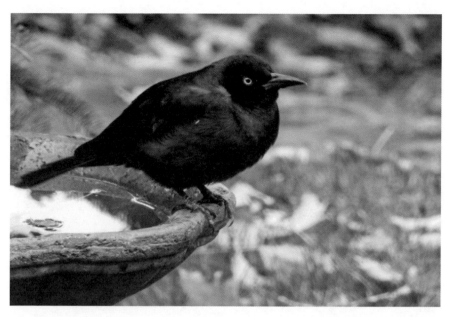

Angry bird at the birdbath

Over time, and with careful observation, you will realize that there is an entire new world for you to learn. I find it fascinating to watch the dynamics between individuals of the same species and between birds of different species. There are dominance rituals playing out that you can observe and learn from and be entertained by. At my feeders I refer to Blue Jays as *Kramer*, the character in the TV sitcom *Seinfeld*, because they make the same crashing, chaotic entrance as he did, usually driving out all the smaller birds. Interspecies interactions can be intriguing to see. I've watched nuthatches and chickadees take peanuts from my feeders to a large maple tree, where they stash them under the bark for later retrieval, only to see them stolen a short time later by a squirrel.

In the first of the following two photos, there are three Baltimore Orioles, a brick-red coloured Orchard Oriole with its back to the camera, as well as a pair of Northern Cardinals canoodling while sharing a seed. Blissful coexistence? A minute later, an epic battle broke out between an Orchard Oriole and Baltimore Oriole, as seen in the second photo. Who needs television when you get this sort of entertainment for free?

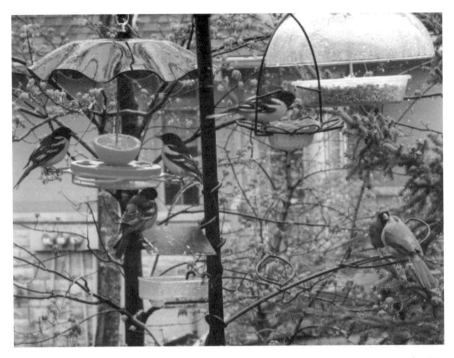

A busy spring day at my feeders

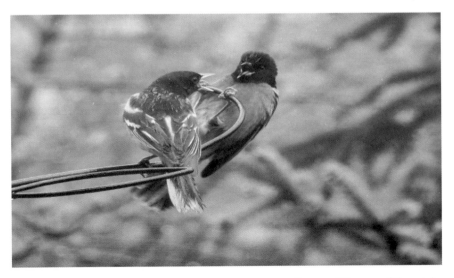

Game on! The war of the orioles

Birds are incredibly tough and endure many hardships. Sometimes I feel that I should be doing more than just feeding them. This photo of two shivering Carolina Wrens, huddling together to stay warm, was taken in early January 2018, on a day that was -20° C. I wanted to invite them inside to warm up.

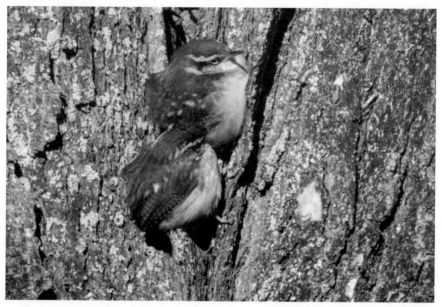

Carolina Wrens toughing it out together

If you are lucky to have birds nesting in or near your yard, it is wonderful to see the parents bringing their youngsters to the feeders once they are old enough to fly. These "fledglings" will often sit on the feeder and squawk for their mom or dad to feed them, even when they look large enough to do so on their own. Here is a photo I took of a father Baltimore Oriole feeding his fledgling.

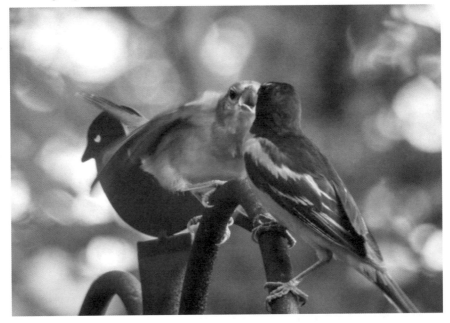

Baltimore Oriole doing dad duty

Evolution is very creative at providing different strategies for repro-duction and raising young. Brown-headed Cowbirds do not build their own nest; they lay eggs in other species' nests and leave it to the host bird to raise their young. This strategy, called nest parasitism, is believed to have evolved when the cowbirds followed herds of bison to catch insects stirred up as they grazed. Because the bison were always on the move from one area to another, the cowbirds couldn't stick around one area long enough to build a nest and raise a family. Whereas most songbirds might lay four to eight eggs in one season (in one or two broods), cowbirds might lay up to thirty-six single eggs a year. The cowbird chick often hatches first and is typically larger than the host young, so they frequently get a disproportionate share of the food brought by the parents and will even smother the smaller birds or kick them out of the nest.

In the following photo, a Chipping Sparrow parent, on the left, is feeding its much larger "baby" Brown-headed Cowbird.

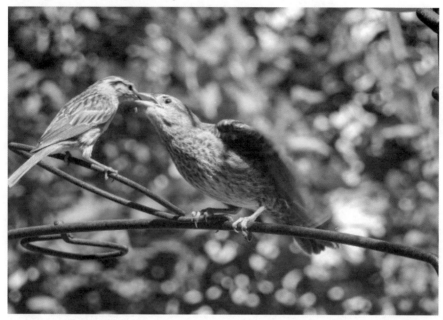

Will you be my mother? Juvenile Brown-headed Cowbird
with Chipping Sparrow parent at my feeders

Although I've spent a fair bit of time discussing backyard bird feeding, I realize that some readers might be living in an apartment and therefore lack a backyard altogether. If your health permits you to take an easy, short outing, just go for a leisurely stroll through your neighbourhood park or cemetery. Quite often, birds are far more concentrated in these small, urban oases than they are out in forests, where they can be scattered over a larger area.

Finally, for those whose health simply doesn't support getting out, or for whatever reason can't watch birds out the window, I recommend you seek out live webcams. There are numerous internet sites that host live video feed from various locations around the world. Nestcams are particularly popular, allowing one to follow raptors such as owls or eagles as they raise their young. Unfortunately, too many folks these days are so removed from the reality of nature that they get overly distressed when seeing bloody carrion being torn apart by raptors to feed their young. In other cases, viewers have watched larger chicks peck a weaker, smaller sibling to death, and the person running the camera will take abuse for letting nature run its course by not intervening. Bald Eagle nestcams are very popular; however, occasionally they have recorded the adults bringing meals to their offspring that upset the viewers. In one infamous case involving a dead cat, the people running the webcam apparently got death threats and had to shut the site down. The people making the threats probably don't give a second thought as to how the steak they enjoy gets to their plate, or to the large number of birds that the cat killed before the tables turned. Nature is indeed "red in tooth and claw."

One interesting webcam is based at the top of the Sheraton Hotel in Hamilton, Ontario, just a few miles from my home. Peregrine Falcons have been successfully breeding here for about 25 years, and the live feed allows one to watch the parents raise their young. I'm not going to recommend any other particular nestcam, as they come and go and a simple internet search will find you plenty. In addition to nestcams, feedercams are very popular. For example, there is a feedercam in Manitouwadge, in northwestern Ontario, that was set up in conjunction with the Cornell Lab of Ornithology (which I will discuss in more detail later) and is being followed in more than 120 countries. There is a website called Bird Feeder Webcams which provides an extensive list of global feeder cams.

8. BEYOND BACKYARD BIRDING

If you are a total birding neophyte, or a "noob," as my son would say, there are numerous resources to aid in identifying various bird species. It doesn't matter if you cannot identify many or any birds. Everyone starts as a beginner, and it certainly isn't something to stress over when you're already ill. You might be pleasantly surprised by how many species you do know, for example the American Robin, the Blue Jay, the Black-capped Chickadee, and the Northern Cardinal. As you learn more, you will gain more confidence and pride in your knowledge. A positive feedback loop happens, and the more you learn, the more you want to learn. Soon, you realize there's a whole world out there waiting for you to experience. One pro tip for beginners, which I learned early on, is that there's no such bird as a "seagull." On an early field trip, I made a comment about a seagull in a farm field and had several birders turn and give me a look; one said, "They're gulls; where's the sea?" There are numerous species of gulls, and many live around freshwater lakes nowhere near the sea. What the layman calls a *seagull* is likely one of two common species, at least here, but could potentially be any one of many different species, which to my eye are all lookalike.

As you learn more, you might wonder why so many of our North American bird names start with *American*—for example, American Robin, American Goldfinch, American Crow, American Redstart, and American Kestrel. This is because the early North American settlers, who mostly originated from the British Isles, noticed birds that reminded them of home but realized they were slightly different. Hence, we have an American Robin, whereas the Robin (also called the European Robin), which resides in the UK and across Europe, is superficially similar looking, but is not even closely related.

Over my first winter of retirement, as I settled in to researching birds and watching my feeders, I discovered that there was a very active Hamilton Naturalists' Club with many knowledgeable members happy to mentor and teach beginning birders. There are no dumb questions. They hold monthly meetings, which I have yet to attend, as they are in the evenings, when my energy is at its lowest. More important to me, they host local field trips.

My first exposure to the club was when I participated in an April 2016 field trip, which I touched on briefly in Chapter 6. I was amazed at how generous the members were with their time and knowledge, patiently tolerating my beginner's questions, with the possible exception of the response to my naive reference to seagulls! I quickly learned that not all birders are as enthused as me over an Eastern Bluebird. I suspect that my gushing over seeing a pair of bluebirds was quite annoying while they were excitedly concentrating on a Sandhill Crane through a scope, a commonplace species to someone from Northern Ontario, where bluebirds are less common. I guess the idea that "one man's junk is another man's treasure" even applies to birding.

I also mentioned in Chapter 6 that during that first field trip I met two experienced birders, Peter Thoem and Barry Coombs, both of whom I name in the Acknowledgments section at the end of the book. Thanks to that initial field trip, I gained two new friends who have mentored me, taken me birding many times, and invited me to participate in a number of bird census outings. When we can't get out birding, we get together for a pub lunch. I never dreamed that I'd make new friends at my age! I can't speak for other countries, but in North American culture, we tend to make most of our friends either in school when we're children or as work colleagues when we enter the work force as young adults. As we age, most people tend to find it harder to meet people and make new friends, and by retirement years, for many it seems that the friend-making part of life is over. I had never anticipated making new friends in my late fifties; certainly not after retirement. Birding has not only made me new friends but has enveloped me in a whole new community I hadn't previously known. I've also met new friends initially via online platforms like Facebook and then subsequently in person while birding, or when my birding friends introduce me to their birding friends. In fact, of my 260 Facebook friends, over half are friends I've met through birding—folks I didn't know at all just a few short years ago! Who would have thought that birding could also be a remedy for the loneliness that can come with illness, aging, and just life in general?

During that field outing I was made aware of a weekly wildflower walk led by a local couple; they hike a different trail every week. I joined up, I'm embarrassed to say, more for my interest in getting to know the local trail systems than in flowers. In fact, on one outing, the group moved on well ahead of me and one other participant as we went crazy photographing a Black-billed Cuckoo.

So, based on my experience, I strongly recommend you seek out any local naturalists' clubs, or failing that, perhaps a photography club, which leads me to another benefit of having participated in that spring field trip. Two individuals separately recommended the Nikon Cool Pix P900 to me. It has a fixed single lens with an incredible 83 times optical zoom. With my Parkinson's-like tremor and mechanical ineptitude, it is the perfect camera for me, as it is light and simple to run. There is no stopping to change lenses or need to fuss with settings, although you can, if you are so inclined. I have met numerous birders who use this so-called "bridge" camera rather than tote around massive lenses and a tripod. While I was writing this book, Nikon released an upgrade, the P1000, with an amazing 125 times optical zoom. Undoubtedly this will lower the price of the P900 and make it even more affordable than it already is.

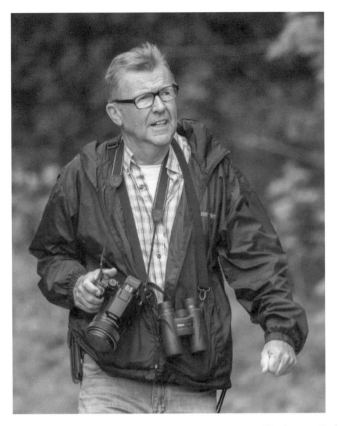

"In the zone" while birding

The Hamilton Naturalists' Club has a Listserv bird alert system. Anyone coming across a bird that will likely be of interest to others is able to send an email that will reach all of the roughly 650 members in real time, or post it on an app called Discord. There is also a similar Ontario-wide Listserv system with about 3,700 members. These alerts often result in numerous birders converging on various hotspots, and as a result, I began to meet more and more like-minded people. Many of them I realized I knew by name, from their alerts to this email system or their Facebook postings to birding sites that we each happened to belong to. As a result, my new network of friends continues to expand by leaps and bounds. Another aspect of this new network that I really enjoy is the fact that these folks with a common passion for birds (and usually for nature in general) come from all walks of life and varying educational levels. During my thirty-five-year career I tended to only socialize with colleagues, so I was in a bit of a bubble.

Many traditional, old-timer birders carry only binoculars ("bins"), while some carry both bins and a camera. When I do carry both, as seen in the previous photo, I utilize a holster that keeps my bins below or to the side of my camera and reduces the strain on my neck. The binoculars I use are Monarch M511, 8 x 42, made by Nikon.

Having a camera with an incredible zoom at my fingertips, I have elected to do most of my birding only with my camera, for a couple of reasons. Firstly, I found it too cumbersome to carry both, and too heavy for my aching body, especially before I bought the holster. Secondly, with the incredible zoom, I could get a pretty good look at a distant bird through the camera. I realize that I miss many birds this way, as it takes longer to get the bird into focus through a camera than through binoculars. But more importantly, as a beginning birder, I often had no idea what bird species I was looking at, so if I could get a photo, I'd take it home and look it up. Gaining this souvenir became a great new challenge, and I found myself striving to get better and better photographs. For me, as an avid collector, building a collection of excellent bird photos is much more exciting now than collecting stamps or rocks and minerals ever was. In fact, I have just sold a considerable portion of my stamp collection and plan to utilize the proceeds for birding trips. I rarely if ever open the stamp books to look at them, whereas I am constantly going through my bird photos. I'm finding more and more birders, especially younger ones, carrying only a camera and not binoculars. It really comes down to personal preference; it is certainly helpful to purchase a decent camera or binoculars, or both.

However, later I will discuss how tensions occasionally arise between birding photographers and birding "purists" who only want to see a bird and couldn't care at all about getting a picture.

It's hard to believe now, but early ornithologists, in the days before binoculars or cameras, would shoot birds so that they could study them in hand. Thankfully, those days are long over. Incidentally, the earlier practice of shooting birds led to some species being named after some obscure feature only visible when up close and personal. For example, the Semipalmated Plover is named for its partially webbed feet, which aren't exactly visible on a wading shorebird!

The next item that I recommend is a good, durable field guide to birds. Any decent bookstore, or store that specializes in bird feeding, such as Wild Birds Unlimited, will have a good selection to choose from. You can't go wrong with big names such as Audubon's, Sibley, Peterson, and Crossley. Some books have broad coverage; for example, books titled "Birds of North America." I recommend you find ones more specific to your particular area, such as Birds of Eastern North America, or Birds of Ontario, so you don't get overwhelmed by dozens of species you're not likely to see anyway. If you believe you have correctly identified a mystery bird using a guide book, do not forget to check its range map; if you are nowhere near its normal range, you likely have misidentified it. Then, if you happen to tell others what you think you saw, the word might spread like wildfire and you could inadvertently be responsible for sending a huge throng of excited birders on a wild goose chase! Birders cannot resist rarities.

Once you progress and get interested in particular types of birds, there are guides that go into great detail on specific families of birds, for example books just on owls, or gulls, or hawks. I recommend a series written by a Canadian, Chris Earley. His titles include *Hawks & Owls of Eastern North America*; *Waterfowl of Eastern North America*; *Sparrows & Finches of the Great Lakes Region & Eastern North America*; and *Warblers of the Great Lakes Region & Eastern North America*. These books aren't just sold in southern Ontario; I have seen them available at the Black Swamp Bird Observatory Shop at Magee Marsh in Ohio.

Being a warbler lover, I bought *The Warbler Guide* by Tom Stephenson and Scott Whittle. It is also available as an app that is so sophisticated that you can manipulate the view of a bird such that you can see what it looks like from the top down, side view, or, as is often the case with warblers, from its underside while it is foraging at the top of a tree.

Another excellent guide for more advanced birders is *Pete Dunne's Essential Field Guide Companion*. Dunne's book has no fancy drawings or photographs. It is all text, but that text is exceptionally descriptive and even at times entertaining. Dunne has suggested that the muted plumage of a Pine Warbler is "roughed out and shabby, a watercolour field sketch of a warbler that the artist never returned to." His description of the stocky Kentucky Warbler is "it is a warbler built to compete in the decathlon." Perhaps the most vivid is his description of the vocalizations of the Blue-winged Warbler; "The first note is higher and often has a zinging electric quality; the second is flatter and sometimes has a flatulent quality."

For my specific area, local expert birder Robert Curry published "*Birds of Hamilton and Surrounding Areas*" in 2006. What makes Curry's book particularly useful is that he compiled all of the historic migration data he could get his hands on and then conducted various statistical analyses with it. Hence, for each migratory bird that breeds here, he gives the median date of spring arrival and fall departure. For birds that we only see passing through on migration, he provides the spring arrival date, spring departure for further north to their summer breeding grounds, fall arrival date, and then fall departure date to their wintering grounds. This data is surprisingly accurate; or perhaps what I should say is that birds are surprisingly consistent as to when they initiate migration. For example, the median arrival date here for Baltimore Orioles is May 3 and fall departure is September 8. In the five years of watching my feeders, the birds have been within one or two days of these dates every year. This data also leads to birders trying to achieve "record dates"; for example, for either the earliest ever spring arrival or latest fall departure. I should mention though, that with climate change, spring arrival dates are trending earlier and earlier.

Younger birders, or more computer-savvy birders, now have their choice of several very reasonably priced apps that they can run on their smart phones, thus mitigating the need to lug a book around. These apps provide descriptions and photos of both adult males and females, as well as juveniles; range maps; and a library of various songs and contact calls that you can play so that you can learn to bird "by ear." Technology changes quickly, and newer apps, websites, and gadgets will continue to appear. The app I currently use is called iBird Pro. It is not expensive, yet very useful. As I write this, Sibley, which has produced a series of excellent bird guide books, has just released an upgraded version of its birding app. In an article titled

"The best birding apps are ones tied to bird guidebooks," Jim Williams reviews and compares a number of birding apps.

Cornell's Lab of Ornithology has a free app you can download called Merlin Bird ID. If you've taken a photo of a "mystery bird," you can load it into Merlin, give it the location and date, and a few seconds later Merlin tells you what it is. It typically gives two or three choices, especially for very similar species, but its first choice is correct about ninety percent of the time. In 2021 a recording capability was added to Merlin, making it the "Shazam" of birding. Once you hit record on the app, a sonogram appears and then quickly the bird is identified. I find this to be an incredibly useful feature.

If you wish to keep a record of the birds you've seen on an outing, it is handy to have a pocket-sized notebook. Rite in the Rain makes good-quality ones, with weatherproofed paper for those less-than-perfect days. Ironically, other than the cover, it is identical to the field notebooks I carried as a geologist. My son gave me one for Father's Day, but given that the apple didn't fall far from the tree, he doctored it up by pasting in a cartoon. I don't know where he found it, but it served a double purpose of being both bird-themed and father-son themed. A juvenile bird and its father are flying together above a road, with junior complaining, "But Dad, I really have to go" and the exasperated parent replying, "All right, all right, there's a car windshield at the next exit!"

The Cornell Lab of Ornithology, based at Cornell University in Ithaca, New York, is in my opinion the premier source for information on birds. Their *All About Birds* website is my go-to resource. Cornell also offers a number of online courses one can subscribe to. I have thoroughly enjoyed and enormously benefited from a number of these courses, taken at my leisure and at a pace that I can handle. Titles include *"Be a Better Birder: Hawk & Raptor Identification Archived Series"*; *"Be a Better Birder: Duck and Waterfowl Identification"*; *"Think Like a Bird: Understanding Bird Behavior"*; *"Spring Field Ornithology—Northeast"*; and *"Warbler Identification."*

One of the key drivers of modern-day birding is eBird, a Cornell initiative that allows birders to post checklists of birds they've seen and search the database for other people's sightings. This initiative is the world's largest citizen-science program, collecting more than 100 million bird observations per year. The resulting database has allowed ornithologists to produce far better range maps for each bird species; they are now dynamic and essentially density maps. Take the Wood Thrush, for example; the following is its range map in traditional format, which does not use this citizen-gathered data. It is simply a fixed map, that doesn't give the viewer any idea if there are "hot spots" within each coloured area where there might be a better chance of seeing a Wood Thrush.

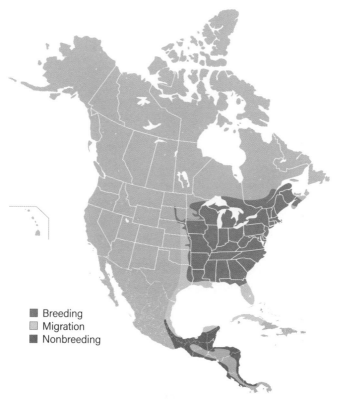

Breeding
Migration
Nonbreeding

Tradtional range map for the Wood Thrush
(Source: Wikipedia – see Notes and References sections)

Compare that map to the new abundance maps eBird can produce based on data collected by "citizen scientist" birders. Now you can see the actual population densities, allowing you to assess the likelihood of seeing one in any given area within the overall range.

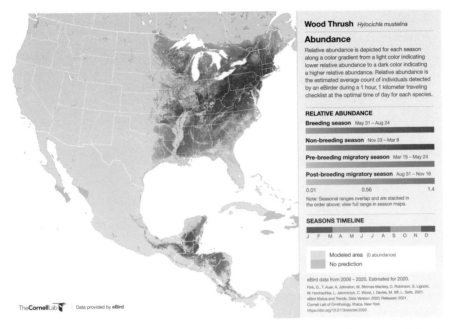

New abundance map for the Wood Thrush
(Source: eBird – see Notes and References sections)

A very helpful feature of eBird is that you can sign up for rare-bird alerts, summarized in daily emails for the geographic region of your choosing. This is a great way to keep tabs on what others are seeing.

I must admit that I have not established a routine of posting my bird sightings on eBird. My reluctance to do so when I first began birding was due to my insecurity in my knowledge; I did not want to post misinformation that might get others excited and send them off on a wild goose chase. Because Lyme gives me anxiety over having any sort of commitments or obligations, I still haven't started, even though I now recognize the vast majority of birds I see. Having to file eBird reports would be stressful to me and make birding feel like work. I feel that I should be contributing, given that I take advantage of it, making queries on either geographical areas that I plan on visiting or on specific species that I'd like to see. I'm thankful there is a vast army of birders out there who don't have such problems and routinely file their observations; I know several sophisticated birders that can do this in real-time as they bird, on a mobile version of the app on their smart phones. For those interested in knowing more about eBird, Cornell provides a free course on how to utilize this amazing program, called eBird Essentials.

In addition to Cornell, there are numerous other excellent bird websites. The *Audubon Guide to North American Birds* is a fantastic resource. Another site I visit frequently is the Boreal Songbird Initiative's *Comprehensive Guide to Boreal Birds,* since so many of my beloved warblers breed in the boreal forests of northern Canada.

While I was working, I had refused family pressure to join Facebook, as I didn't want my private life exposed to shareholders of my company, especially if they were mad at me for the share price! But once I retired, I joined and learned that, not only was it a great way to reconnect with extended family such as cousins and nieces and nephews, it opened up an entire new facet of birding to me. There are numerous fantastic Facebook bird groups—some dedicated to specific areas or specific families of birds, some global, some to help with bird identification, and some for rare bird alerts. It took me a while to sift through and find the best ones. Unfortunately, there are many that are a waste of time; if I see one that captions every photo "rate this bird for cuteness from one to ten," I'm out of there. Such sites frequently have photos that are clearly doctored and so altered with Photoshop that the birds are obviously in false colours.

I have compiled a list of a few of the many birding Facebook groups that I belong to and recommend, which is provided in the *Resources* section (Appendix B) near the end of this book. Most of these are closed groups, which you must request permission to join (which only requires the click of a button, at least to inquire if not gain access). Given the ephemeral nature of Facebook groups and other internet content, I hope these suggestions will at least inspire to you search for groups and pages, or any digital resource, to support your birding passion at whatever time you may be reading this book. As of this writing, the *Algoma District Birding* group is run by a very knowledgeable young naturalist and expert birder by the name of Carter Dorscht. Both my hometown of Sault Ste. Marie and our family cottages on Bright Lake are in the Algoma District in northern Ontario. The *Birds, Blooms, Beasts, Bugs and Butterflies* site is run by a friend of mine, Barb Canney, from Waterdown, Ontario. Barb makes this site a lot of fun and in just a few years has driven the membership from a handful of personal friends to 7,800 worldwide members. Finally, the *Ontario Bird Photography* group was set up by my good friend and birder-photographer extraordinaire Bill McDonald.

Rather than merely posting photos on Facebook, some birders choose to post on a Flickr page or on their own blog; some on multiple media. Peter Thoem, Barry Coombs, and Bill McDonald all have blogs that I recommend and have listed in the *Resources* section. An exceptional blog is run by my friend Andrew Mactavish. Andrew is not only an amazing photographer; he is highly knowledgeable and provides very informative, educational narratives to accompany his first-class photos. Other new friends who post fantastic photos on Flickr include Steve Rossi, Randy Droniuk, and Ed O'Connor. Doug Ward is an exceptional photographer; his photos can be seen on his Facebook page. Again, please see the *Resources* section for links to their sites. I would like to add a universal apology to innumerable other friends whom I haven't explicitly named here who are excellent birders and/or photographers as well.

If you are lucky enough to have a nearby university or arboretum that might offer courses, I'd suggest you take advantage of them. I've mentioned Chris Earley as a great author of birding books. He is also the most inspirational, motivating lecturer you could ever find. Chris's day job is as Interpretive Biologist and Education Coordinator at the University of Guelph Arboretum, where I've taken two of his courses, on owls and warblers.

Another way to get exposed to birding and learn more is to visit a banding station, if you should have one close to you. I'm blessed in having two nearby: one at Long Point on Lake Erie, run by Birds Canada (a Canadian federal government agency) and another at Ruthven, which is about a half-hour drive from my house. In the fall, Ruthven conducts Northern Saw-whet Owl banding, and when we visited during an evening open house, we were thrilled to see that they had caught two. However, shortly thereafter they had a record night of eighteen captured and banded. I've included a photo of a Saw-whet taken after it was assessed and banded, prior to being released.

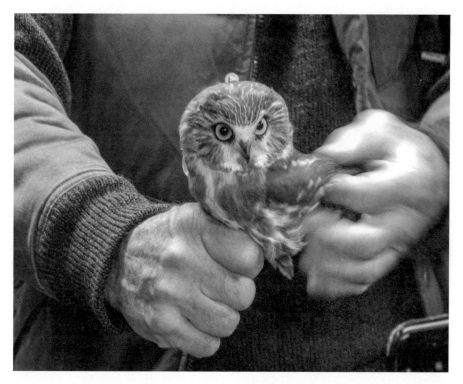

Northern Saw-whet Owl about to be banded

The social media platform *Twitter* has become a modern-day way of "following" and hearing the thoughts of interesting birders, photographers, naturalists, and experts. I follow dozens, far too numerous to mention all of them. Twitter handles for those I'm about to discuss can be found in the *Resources* section. Birders who currently post wonderful photos that have been taken respectfully (without unduly stressing or harassing the bird) include Maranda Mink, Mali, and Jim Pottkotter. The raw, sheer excitement and joy of encountering and photographing birds comes through loud and clear in their tweets.

On the lighter side, I love following the twitter account of Karl Mechem, who tweets using the handle *@TheIneptBirder*. He plays up his ability to take pathetically bad photos of birds, such as the butt ends of birds flying away, pictures out of focus, or quivering branches where the bird just was. Very entertaining, and something I think most of us can relate to.

I have built an entire library of bird books over the past three years; however, certain ones stand out head and shoulders above the rest. A list with a brief description of recommended books can be found in the *Resources* section.

There are also several excellent birding videos that I've bought and can strongly recommend. The Great Courses released *The National Geographic Guide to Birding in North America*, hosted by James Currie. This four CD set contains twenty-four half-hour lessons. For those delving in a bit deeper, Michael Male and Judy Fieth put out two videos called *Watching Sparrows* and *Watching Warblers*.

PBS produced an excellent DVD called *Owl Power*; it can be found on Amazon. In my experience, most people are fascinated by owls, particularly children. Perhaps it is the influence of Harry Potter. I've learned that when giving my library bird talks, I need to keep owls to the end. Otherwise, I peak too soon and anything I say after showing owl photos is anticlimactic.

For anyone interested in learning bird songs and therefore gaining the ability to bird by ear, an application called Larkwire is an absolute must. This interactive, educational yet entertaining program makes learning fun by allowing you to test your knowledge of bird songs at different levels of difficulty. I know many birders who have the most amazing ability to identify birds by ear alone. I have a hearing impairment that has been exacerbated by Lyme, increasing my tinnitus to the point I don't hear well and have a very hard time differentiating the subtle variations in songs of related birds, such as warblers. However, even I can probably recognize fifty or more species by song alone. I bet the average person knows far more bird songs than they are consciously aware of. For example, if you live in North America, you most likely are familiar with the calls or songs of the American Robin, the American Crow, the Blue Jay, the Northern Cardinal and the Black-capped Chickadee, its onomatopoeic name based on its emphatic chick-a-dee-dee-dee call. For anyone who is visually impaired and interested in the benefits of birding, don't feel left out, as you might find birding by ear very enjoyable. I suggest you refer to an article titled *"Birding Blind: Open Your Ears to the Amazing World of Bird Sounds"* by Trevor Attenberg.

If your health does permit you to do more than backyard bird, where do you start? Birders are a strange lot. We love garbage dumps, sewage lagoons, water treatment plants, and cemeteries! Cemeteries provide excellent habitat for many different species of birds, and quite often, in particular for owls. Large, mature trees provide roosting spots from which to look out over vast open areas for prey animals such as mice, voles, and smaller birds. A local cemetery close to my home is host to two Eastern Screech-Owls. However, they are so well known that there have been conflicts between birders and people paying homage to loved ones. Etiquette and respect are obviously much needed to bird in a cemetery.

Isolated woodlots and parks along the shores of the Great Lakes are excellent migrant "traps"—if the birds have flown across the open water, they are exhausted and hungry and can become very concentrated in such areas. Add a rainstorm that grounds the birds during migration, and these so called "fallouts" can be a birder's paradise. In southern Ontario such areas include Point Pelee Provincial Park, Rondeau Provincial Park, Long Point, Edgelake in Stoney Creek, and Sedgewick Forest in Oakville. If you recall the map I included earlier, Point Pelee and Long Point provide migrating birds shortcuts across Lake Erie. Point Pelee is internationally famous for birders and during peak migration in early to mid-May is exceptionally busy.

Sedgewick is a woodlot adjacent to a sewage treatment plant. The warm water creates a microclimate and results in midges and other insects hatching year-round, providing plenty of food for warblers, kinglets, and other bird species. Unfortunately, every year a few individual birds get lulled into staying put and not migrating as they should, and when a really cold snap comes, they may not survive it. Other sewage lagoons and settling ponds can be a great place for viewing gulls and shorebirds, provided the appropriate governing body allows access.

A brief time spent searching the internet, especially eBird, will introduce you to the bird species that you might encounter in an area you plan to visit. At the same time, you can find out where the hot spots are, such as parks, birding trails, nature reserves and conservation areas.

If you are up to traveling to a new spot, say a Caribbean vacation, and are keen to do some birding, I strongly recommend you check out the *Birding Pal* website. The cost is only $10 annually, and the site can connect you with a local birder who will guide you. These are usually volunteers who are simply happy to share their knowledge and show off their local birds. You don't have to pay your birding pal, but you should pick up all the expenses such as gas, meals, or entrance fees into parks. It is a fantastic concept for those on a busy vacation or business trip who might have a spare day or even just a few hours to get out and do some birding.

9. EVEN BIRDING HAS POLITICS

I quickly learned that birding is as subject to political conflicts as any other field. Earlier I alluded to a controversy that exists between birders and photographers. Birding "purists" just want to see the bird and don't care about getting a photograph of it. Some of them look down on bird photographers with disdain, and sometimes for good reason. By bird photographers, I'm not referring to people like myself who bird with cameras, but rather, photographers who are there only to get a "money shot," whether for personal satisfaction or commercial use. Obviously, this does not apply to all photographers, but some may seek an awesome shot at the expense of the bird, for example by getting too close and stressing it, or flushing it out of its hiding spot, thus exposing it to possible predation. The ultimate in controversy is baiting owls. Many spectacular face-on photos of an owl swooping in to catch its prey have been staged, with store-bought mice thrown out or even pinned down, to entice the owl. This habituates the owls to people and can lead them to being hit and killed by cars along a roadside when baited.

I find myself to be a combination birding enthusiast and bird photographer. I did not set out to collect bird photos. As I mentioned earlier, birding with a camera was the only way I could determine what I was looking at when I first started birding, by capturing an image I could later research. Even though I am far more knowledgeable now and can usually identify the birds I see in the field, I continue to use a camera. As my photography skills have developed, I find myself taking great pride in capturing a beautiful photograph. I have been making calendars with my bird photos as Christmas gifts for a few years now. However, I still consider myself primarily a birder, not a photographer. The sheer thrill of seeing a bird is good enough for me, but I'm even happier if I "capture" it with a great photo.

My second revelation about birding politics was to discover how competitive birding can be. Birders love to keep lists; these can range from a backyard list, to a county, province or state list, a year list, a life list, or even a seasonal list. For example, a rarity on a winter list might be a very common summer resident, but because it hasn't migrated as it should have, it is an exciting rarity to add to the list; it is a rarity in time, not location. This passion for having the most species on a list leads a number of very competitive birders to do a "Big Year": to go all-out in a certain region and try to set a record for the most bird species seen in one calendar year. The competitive nature of these Big Years was captured hilariously (or mocked?) in the 2011 movie *The Big Year*, starring Owen Wilson, Steve Martin, and Jack Black. I previously mentioned the entertaining "Inept Birder" who tweets bad photos frequently; keeping with his sense of humour, he announced in 2019 that he was doing a "Biggish" Year.

In 2015, a young American birder named Noah Strycker aimed to set the world record for a Big Year, not for a state or region, but for the entire planet. There are roughly 10,000 species of birds in the world; the exact number is in flux, thanks in part to advances in genetic testing. DNA is showing that some birds considered separate species should actually be lumped together as one; conversely, other birds previously lumped as one species are being split into two or more. At any rate, Strycker set a goal to see at least 5,000 species in 2015, or roughly half of the world's birds. He ended up seeing 6,042. He wrote an entertaining book about his adventures called *Birding without Borders*; I highly recommend it. Organizing his year-long adventure required an immense amount of planning in order to maximize bird species seen in minimal time, with the least amount of travel and backtracking. Closer to home, young birder and naturalist Jeremy Bensette did a Big Year in 2017 in the province of Ontario. He set a new Ontario record, with 346 species seen.

Perhaps it was inevitable in this digital era: as I was writing this book, someone came up with the concept of *"Fantasy Birding."* It is loosely based on Fantasy Sports, where armchair athletes can draft and trade various players and then compete against one another using those players' real-life statistics to score points. Fantasy Birding is like doing a Big Year from the comfort of home. Each day you choose a location to visit and bird, using variables such as weather forecasts and recent sightings in eBird to guide your planning. You then earn points for all the birds observed and reported in eBird near your chosen location. The challenge is to find a balance between birding reliable hot spots and chasing rarities.

As competitive as I am, rather than seeking the longest checklist, I get my satisfaction from seeing new species and capturing a great photo to be proud of. I can then spend hours labeling, sorting, and filing my photos and organizing them.

I mentioned earlier that the Hamilton Naturalists' Club has an email and app "hot line" where folks will post rare sightings in real time and that there is another one for the entire province of Ontario. Other sources post sightings via Twitter, Facebook or WhatsApp. By following the emails and tweets (appropriately enough) about bird sightings at various locations, I've learned all the local hot spots of where to go and what to expect. Many avid listers will "chase", or "twitch" in British parlance, every rare bird posting. From my perspective some of these folks seem to be driven more by their desire to have the largest list rather than the joy of actually seeing the bird. I can't be bothered to chase birds, with the few odd exceptions. With my luck, I could drive several hours and the bird will have moved on; they do, after all, have wings. Just in the past year or so I've known folks in my area to have driven 975 kilometres to Wawa, Ontario to see a wayward bird from Mexico, and 1,440 kilometres to northern New Brunswick for a bird from Europe. A hummingbird from the west coast of North America showed up at a feeder in southern Ontario, and about 800 birders made the trek to see it.

I admit, though, that if there is a bird that everyone is seeing and I haven't "chased" it, I occasionally suffer from the condition known as FOMO—fear of missing out. A couple of years ago, a Yellow-headed Blackbird, very uncommon for my area, was reported in the marshy reeds around a storm drainage pond only about a twenty-minute drive from my house. The alert came out about 5 p.m., and I had just awakened from my afternoon nap and was too groggy to go. I figured since it was late in the day, the bird would be there the next morning. Wrong. There were about twenty-five other birders there early the next morning, but no Yellow-headed Blackbird. Numerous birders, including a few friends, posted great photos on Facebook from the evening before. I was crippled with FOMO! I turned this disappointment into motivation; when I planned a birding trip through Michigan for the next spring, I included a destination well known for these blackbirds and was rewarded with a "lifer"—a species I was seeing for the first time. Birders who are listing enthusiasts would want this bird on their Ontario list, as it would be rare; I was just happy to see it within its normal range and be able to add it to my life list.

Birding and checklists are not just a North American passion. On January 11, 2019, a European Robin showed up on the grounds of the Beijing Zoo; the blog *Birding Beijing* has a photo showing a crowd of birders estimated at over 200, with an impressive array of cameras all poised to capture a photo. Clearly, there is a bit of interest in birding in China as well! They joked that the robin was a "Brexit refugee."

10. WHY I LOVE BIRDING

Once I was forced to retire thanks to Lyme, I reconciled myself to living with a chronic disease that causes fatigue, muscle and joint pain, and neuropathy that moved beyond peripheral right to my body core. I couldn't sit in one position for more than a minute or two before my butt would go to "sleep" and get that annoying pins-and-needles sensation.

However, I have discovered that I can park these sensations by focusing on birds. So how does this obsession of mine, being a birder, help my health? In a nutshell, it provides me with fresh air, exercise, mental calming, a new hobby I am passionate about, the impetus to learn new things, and camaraderie with new friends; all of which have been therapeutic to my health.

In my youth I was a small game hunter, which I could never do now. Birding brings back the same excitement of tracking and stalking, but without killing anything. The thrill of spotting a rare bird, or a lifer, gets the adrenalin flowing. I have blown many a photograph because I was literally trembling with excitement; I am not good at curbing my enthusiasm if the bird is a lifer or one of my favourite warblers. The important thing, however, is that when I am in such an excited state, I am totally oblivious of my aching body.

Birding challenges my sense of observation, as the loudest singing bird may be smaller than a chickadee and hidden in a tree seventy-five feet up. Hearing a bird singing, patiently waiting for it to reveal itself, and then making an identification, can be exhilarating. And while I'm doing so, it makes me forget about my pains.

I have always kept myself very busy and have always been on the go, carrying out numerous projects such as the bird book which I wrote for my own benefit, writing two in-depth (maternal and paternal) family histories, and writing an entire volume detailing my mineral exploration adventures. Being hyper is something I inherited from my father; it is a family trait. An aunt married to one of my dad's brothers famously once said, "Bells don't get ulcers, they give them!" Birding requires me to be more patient than my normal self, waiting to see an elusive bird, or to get that perfect photo. A hobby that encourages slowing down and calmness has certainly been good for me.

I truly believe there is nothing more therapeutic than being out in nature, spending hours in fresh air in the outdoors, soaking up all the sights, sounds, and smells that nature offers (except of course, the sewage treatment plants that I previously recommended). I explained earlier that backyard birding can be satisfying and helpful to your health, but actually being out in the fresh air and in nature adds another whole level of therapy to your healing.

Another obvious benefit of birding in the outdoors is that I get huge amounts of exercise, which helps me to battle Lyme. I believe that pushing your body to its limits, no matter what those limits might be, is beneficial. It is not uncommon for me to walk three to five kilometers in a day when I am birding—a far cry from just a few years ago, when walking a few hundred metres with the aid of a cane was exhausting. In that zone where I feel peaceful and deeply focused on birds (and therefore not on my symptoms), walking this far does not feel like hard work; I am simply pursuing my passion in a dreamlike trance, and all this exercise is a fantastic bonus that I hardly notice myself doing. Something else worth mentioning is that, as far as having a hobby that provides exercise goes, birding is a relatively safe one. Walking is self-paced, and if you do happen to require the aid of a cane, walker, wheelchair, or any other mobility support device, it will not impede your ability to engage in some level of birding. The degree to which you might immerse yourself in the natural world is also highly variable and up to you: you might travel to a faraway destination to seek birds in a particular wild area, such as a jungle or old-growth forest; you might hike along a local trail; or you might simply look out of your window from your own home! All of these are examples of birding. You may choose what feels safe and satisfying to you. For many, birding is a safer method of exercise than most, especially for those who are elderly, disabled, injured, or convalescing from illness. It is a highly adaptable hobby.

Another collateral benefit to birding for me is that I am slowly developing a new skill: photography. I realize that many birders aren't interested in taking photos and are content to carry just binoculars. For me, there is a sense of pride and accomplishment in learning to capture a good photo, especially if the subject is an elusive, quick-moving bird such as a warbler or kinglet. It is even good for my Lyme-damaged psyche and ego to get "likes" for my photos on Facebook and applause when giving a bird talk, showing off my photos. Granted, many people fall into the trap of basing their self-worth on the approval of others, and that is not healthy either. But the social anxiety spurred on by Lyme and which frequently keeps me away from social settings has benefited from the boost that a little online attention can garner from the comfort and safety of my own home.

I have mentioned earlier that I have been a collector since a young age, including rocks and minerals, stamps, and moths and butterflies. Birding satisfies this obsessive compulsion, as I now strive to "collect birds" by seeing and photographing every species possible. I have found an interesting similarity between collecting bird photos and my previous passion of collecting rock and mineral specimens. When I look back at bird photos I've taken in the past, I often instantly recall the occasion, the location, even the weather at the time of the photo. Likewise, many rock samples in my collection bring back memories of the weather, the tough slog (or not) to get to that location, and sometimes a vivid image of the outcrop I collected them from.

Another of my obsessive-compulsive quirks is organization; my family often jokingly asked when I was going to alphabetize my refrigerator contents. Given that on a birding outing I routinely shoot several hundred photos, there is a lot of organization required in labeling them, with respect to species, location, and date. I keep Excel spreadsheets to track what species I've seen, which I've photographed, or need a better photo of. Many birders utilize functions within eBird to keep themselves organized with their bird lists. Unlike the compulsive listers I described earlier, I only keep a life list, which currently stands at 462 species, and a yard list, which is at 95 species. My yard list would be considerably larger if I was better at identifying birds on the wing; numerous species of gulls, waterfowl, and raptors often fly over my house, but I can't be positive of their identities. You can be as organized (or not) as you'd like to be with how you approach birding, but for those like me who enjoy projects and like to make things just so, there is plenty of this type of work to be found in this hobby, which I find to be very satisfying.

Birding tests my scientific knowledge as I learn to identify species both visually and by ear; I have transitioned from being a professional geologist to an amateur ornithologist. Like any science, the more you learn, the more you realize just how little you know. In this regard, birding also keeps one humble, frequently *very* humble! Just when I think I'm getting good at identifying birds, one will stump me. Even highly experienced birders don't always get it right.

As I've previously discussed, birding has introduced me to an entire new sphere of like-minded folks with whom I enjoy sharing my new passion. Having said that, with all due respect to so many new friends who have been generous with their time and knowledge in mentoring me, I do prefer to do most of my birding on my own. This is nothing personal against any of them. Rather, it is a function of my Lyme that I get stressed by having to conform to anyone else's agenda or timing. On my own, I can spend as much or as little time as I want on any given bird, either by staying put and soaking it in or deciding I've had enough and moving on. I prefer the freedom to follow my whims, and if I "hit the wall" and need to call it a day, I don't have to ruin anyone else's plans. I do try to resist these feelings when I can, as I know that whenever I'm out birding with friends, I will not only have fun but learn new things from them. Also, the shared joy of seeing a rare bird with a friend is a real bonding experience.

I am not a fan of birding in a large group, particularly in congested spring migration hot spots such as Point Pelee or Magee Marsh in Ohio. My anxiety gets triggered if I hear the rapid-fire clicks of dozens of cameras shooting at once, like paparazzi on a red carpet. If I can't see the bird that they're photographing, or can't get it in focus, birding FOMO hits me. I far prefer to be on my own.

I might set out in anticipation of seeing a particular bird species (my "target bird") that has been reported in a certain location. But invariably, there is a surprise. I might get a fantastic look at a bird I wasn't expecting, or get to observe some interesting behaviour interaction between individuals or species, or see something that is new and exciting and above and beyond the expectation that I had. It's like the old saying about lotteries: "If you don't play, you can't win." Well, if you don't get out there and into nature, you don't know what you might have missed. And it might have been incredible: the birding equivalent of those awesome spontaneous parties you've attended that were way better than long-planned and anticipated events. If you are a "lister," perhaps you found something new for your bird list, a lifer, which becomes harder to get as you become more experienced. Or maybe it was a bird you've seen many times, but never in that location, or never before posing in the open, offering you the best photographic opportunity ever. Whatever floats your boat, getting out there will almost always deliver a pleasant surprise; as my friend Peter Thoem refers to them, "My Bird of the Day."

I earlier discussed my interaction with a lady who attended one of my bird talks and had wanted to see a bluebird. Sharing the experience of seeing birds is very satisfying, and I find great joy in introducing others to birds. However, I am fully aware that I can be a bit much in my exuberance for birds, and apparently, I am not the only birder guilty of this. I once saw a meme on a Facebook birding page showing a traditional "swear jar" with a few coins in the bottom of it, and next to it, a jar completely full of money labeled, "Telling people about birds when I wasn't asked jar."

Another thing about birding that appeals to me is the homework, research, and organizing required to put together a trip. This might not sound like fun to most people, but perhaps I enjoy it as it reminds me of the preparation required before I went on my multi-country, often multi-continent business trips. I'd arrange meetings with potential joint venture partners and government officials, along with planned project site visits with my own staff, and lay out detailed logistics to maximize my time and efficiency. Organizing such trips could take weeks to pull together. Now, I find I'm doing the same thing with birding. I research bird sightings using the various tools I've mentioned, such as eBird, and then put together an itinerary of destinations, driving times, hotels, and so on. I don't miss work and wouldn't want it back, now that I am so passionately hooked on birding, but the similarities in organizing trips is an interesting flashback that I enjoy. I do have one major regret about my extensive travel history. Although always interested in and aware of nature around me, I was not an addicted birder on all of those trips and missed many unique opportunities that could never be replicated. Not that I would have had much time to chase birds on those busy trips, but still: my life list could have been three or four times what it is now.

Finally, I love that birding fills me with such eager anticipation as I look forward to the arrival of the next "birding season." It is a year-round hobby that is ever changing, month to month. There is an annual, predictable cyclicity to the ebb and flow of birds; a rhythm that demarks the passage of time. Each birding season brings new birds, new targets, and new places to focus one's energy and time. For most birders, spring is the most beloved time of the year, when songbirds return from their southern wintering grounds to either stay and breed in our neighbourhood or pass through on their way to summer homes farther north. Although where I live some spring migrants, such as Red-winged Blackbirds, can arrive as early as late February or early March, the real action is from late April to late May, when there is wave after wave, pulse after pulse, of my favourite birds returning. Birders routinely check overnight wind forecasts, knowing that southerly winds are favourable for northward-bound migrants, and every morning there is a chance to see beautiful new migrants who arrived overnight. Spring is when the males are dressed in their finest clothing, showcasing their beautiful breeding plumages in hopes of seducing a mate.

The slowest months of the year for birding are actually the summer months. The bird world seems to go quiet; there is less singing and fewer birds at the feeder. Of course, it is not actually quiet in terms of bird activity; they are sitting on eggs and raising their young. Come mid- to late summer, suddenly there are parent birds coming to the feeders with their fledglings. At the same time, as I watch these juvenile songbirds grow up, a new birding season begins: here in Southern Ontario, shorebird fall migration begins in late July, with the arrival of birds such as sandpipers and plovers, who have spent their summers on the shores of James and Hudson Bay, and some even farther north on the Arctic islands.

In mid- to late August, fall migration begins in earnest for the songbirds, and once again, we are inundated with my favourite birds. Many species have now exchanged their breeding plumage for the duller, earth-toned colourings of fall, which can make them harder to identify. I will touch on this in the next chapter when I discuss birding challenges. On the other hand, there are far more birds migrating south in the fall than there are birds migrating north in the spring; in the fall, both the adults and their recently hatched offspring are travelling. In addition, younger birds making their first migration trip are more apt to stray and end up off course; so in the fall there are not only more individual birds, but a greater chance of spotting a rarity.

As we settle into winter, owl season dawns, then duck season, and then finally we loop back around to spring migration again. The earth has made another lap around the sun, the cyclicity of the birds has continued like clockwork, and birders eagerly anticipate each new phase of this amazing journey.

Although I am in awe of all birds, I find that my main love is passerines, commonly referred to as songbirds or perching birds, and the prettier, the better. I know many birders that get thoroughly excited at identifying gulls, all of which are various shades of white, gray, and black. To compound the challenge, gulls typically exhibit a slightly different colour scheme every year until they reach adulthood after several years. Sorry, but they just don't do anything for me. I admit I prefer pretty birds; does that make me a superficial birder?

Below are some of my photos of a few of my favourite things. Of all the various families of birds, warblers are my favourites. They are small, beautiful, and hyperactive; when you try to photograph them you realize their name should be spelled "war-blur!" I am including these photos with the hope of enticing readers to get as excited about birds as I do. And they can all be seen in southern Ontario; some only during migration, as they travel further north to their breeding grounds in the boreal forest, or on their way south to their wintering grounds, which range from the southern USA to Colombia in South America. How could you not love these? Unfortunately, these are not birds that you will see at your feeders, as warblers are insect eaters.

One of the most beautiful warblers, and most coveted by birders, is the Golden-winged Warbler. I was exceptionally pleased to capture this beauty sitting still for a few seconds.

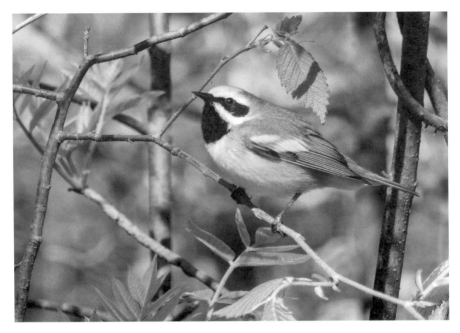

The breathtaking Golden-winged Warbler

The Black-and-white Warbler is like a miniature zebra with wings. They are extremely common around our family cottages in northern Ontario, where I delight in watching them forage for insects by hopping along branches and trunks of trees, reminiscent of a nuthatch.

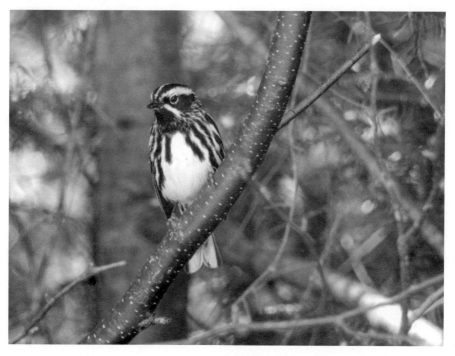

The Black-and-white Warbler, a zebra with wings

The Mourning Warbler gets its name from its black bib, resembling funeral attire. I am very lucky to have several breeding pairs within a few kilometres of my house in Ancaster.

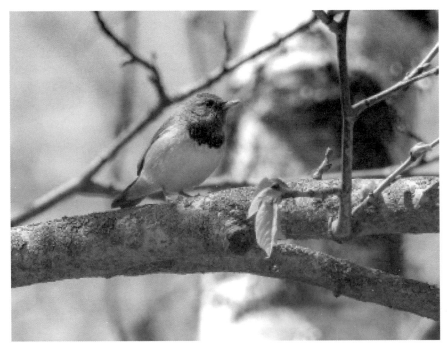

A Mourning Warbler

The Cape May Warbler, shown in the next photo, got its name because the first one ever identified was seen at Cape May, New Jersey. However, at Cape May they are only migrants, and one wasn't seen there again for a century after the first sighting! Mind you, it is not unusual for birds to receive inappropriate names without it being understood until years later that the name is in fact not appropriate. The Palm Warbler may have been first seen in a palm tree on its wintering grounds, but it breeds in boreal forests and even sub-tundra terrain of northern Canada.

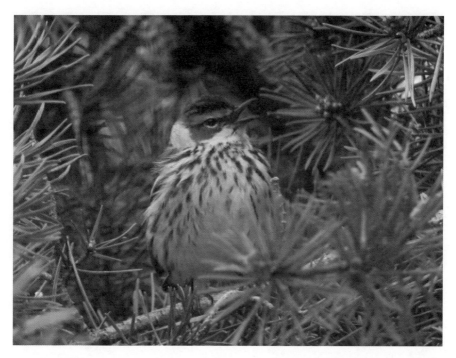

The poorly named Cape May Warbler

When I took his warbler course, Chris Earley referred to the Northern Parula as the "Sunset Warbler", which is a pretty good description given the explosion of colours on its breast.

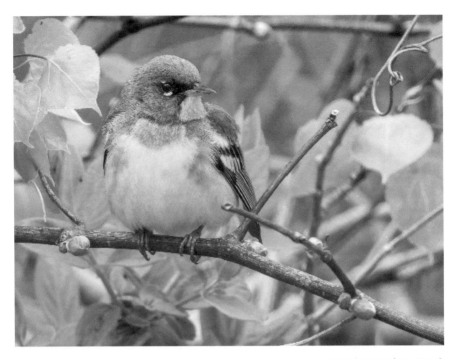

A stunning Northern Parula

The Magnolia Warbler is another warbler with an unfortunate name; the first one identified happened to be sitting in a magnolia tree, which again would only occur during migration, as they breed in northern forests and overwinter in Mexico and Central America, neither of which location is home to magnolia trees. I love the contrast between the bold black stripes and the bright yellow breast.

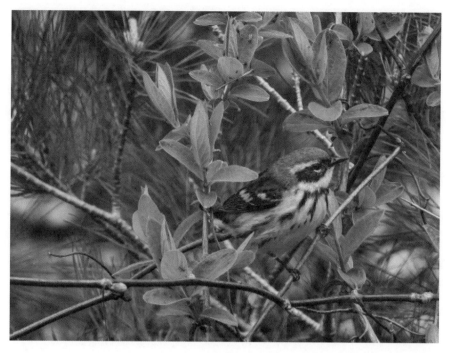

Another poorly named bird, the Magnolia Warbler

The Blackburnian Warbler is, in my opinion, one of the most stunning warblers—the flaming orange of the males' throat and breast is beautifully complemented by its black facial pattern. I was shocked to discover that these gorgeous birds breed right next to our family cottages. I'm embarrassed that I was oblivious to them as a young lad spending his summers there. However, this again exemplifies how discreet they can be. If you don't know what you're looking for, or don't make a point of looking at all, they are easy to miss, as the orange isn't obvious when they are flitting about in the shadows.

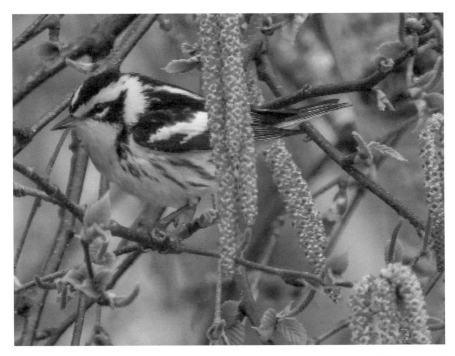

A Blackburnian Warbler, nicknamed "flame throat"

The Canada Warbler is probably tied with the Blackburnian as my favourite; that bold "necklace" and white eyering are spectacular.

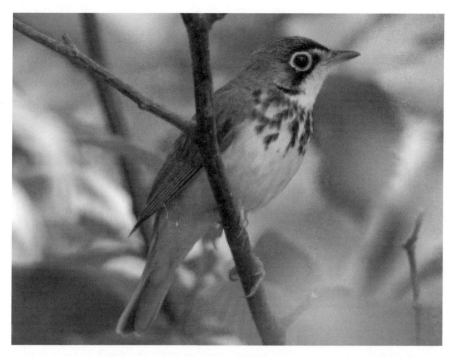

A Canada Warbler seen near our family cottages in Algoma District, Ontario

I could go on and on with warblers; there are about fifty species that breed in the continental USA and Canada, of which about thirty-three are known to breed in Ontario. I will reluctantly end my discussion of warblers with photos of a Black-throated Green Warbler, a bird whose name is longer than itself, and a Chestnut-sided Warbler.

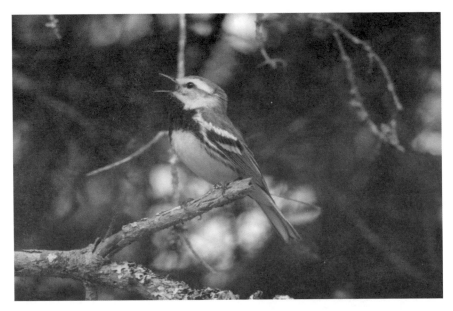

A singing Black-throated Green Warbler

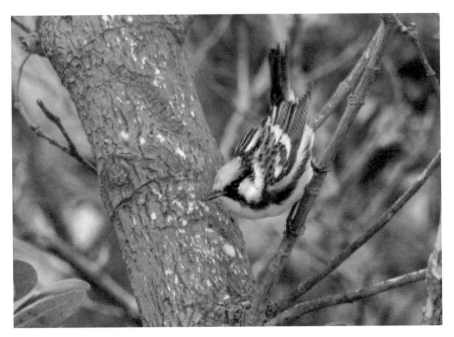

Chestnut-sided Warbler striking a jaunty pose

Although warblers are my favourites, I am always in awe when I see an Eastern Bluebird, one of my favourite birds that is not a warbler, and hence the species I chose for my daughter to paint for the cover. I think I like them even more knowing that I could help the lady who attended one of my library talks to achieve her dream of seeing one. Bluebirds are members of the thrush family, as is the American Robin.

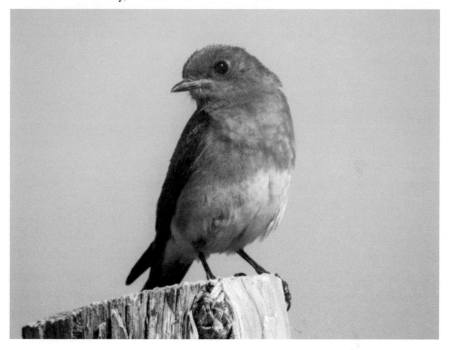

A stunning Eastern Bluebird

I could fill an entire book with photos of my favourite birds, but I will finish with a Ruby-Crowned Kinglet. Smaller than warblers and even more hyper, kinglets are so difficult to photograph that getting a photo of one in focus has been described as akin to "shooting popcorn."

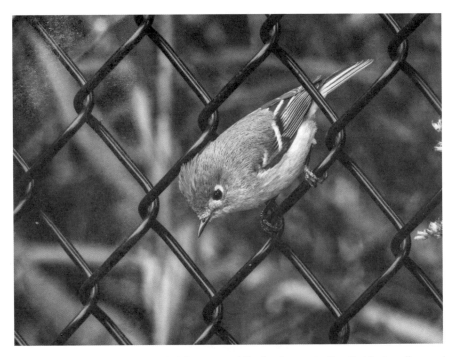

A Ruby-crowned Kinglet demonstrating that he is well-named

I thought it would be appropriate to conclude this chapter on why I love birding by referencing a tweet I happened to come across. On September 22, 2019, Tina Survilla Lindell, quoting a birder whom she had met, tweeted: *"There's no cure. Birdwatching is terminal. When you get it, you got it for life."* I couldn't have said it better myself.

11. BIRDING CHALLENGES

One of the first challenges a novice birder might encounter is the lingo. Like NASA, birders use a number of acronyms that are cryptic until explained. One is "FOY," short for First of the Year. As an example, someone might post a photo of "my FOY Purple Finch." When trying to identify birds, it is recommended that you go with GISS. What's that? General Impression of Size and Shape. Birding code for using gut instinct.

Birders constantly use two phrases that drive me crazy. They are "it was just here" and "you should have been here ten minutes ago!" I have often joked that if I ever wrote a bird book one of these two expressions would be the title of the book. As Maxwell Smart used to say in the 1960s sitcom *Get Smart*, "Missed it by that much!" This is why I tend to not "chase" hot birds of the day. Invariably I arrive to a throng of birders and hear one or both of those expressions. On the bright side, other birding expressions that are appreciated include "nice find" and "well captured," when you manage to get an awesome photo.

Every birder has his or her "nemesis bird." That's a species that you're dying to see; it might be the lifer you've been longing for. Lots of other folks have "got him," but you just keep "dipping" on him. In birding lingo, to *dip* on a bird means you failed to see it, even when many others had reported its presence at a certain location. Once again, birding FOMO strikes! Peter Thoem refers to target birds that he fails to find as "a bird for another day." That nicely sums it up. On the other hand, that also sums up life. If it was all easy and there were no challenges left, life would get pretty boring. I have to keep reminding myself that if it were not for the challenge of Lyme, I would not have become the passionate birder I am today. This makes me think of the old adage, "What doesn't kill you makes you stronger." I had taken this saying to heart after successful surgery for prostate cancer in 2007. Just like my prostate cancer, Lyme didn't kill me, but it has challenged me tremendously, teaching me so much along the way, and has opened me up to an entirely new world. This new world of birding and my passion for it have certainly made me stronger and happier.

Since I began seriously birding in 2016, I have had two nemesis birds: Bohemian Waxwings and Long-eared Owls. I don't even want to think of how many trips I took and how many miles I drove in search of these birds, only to be denied and dip on them repeatedly. The winter of 2019 finally brought me success with both—here is a photo I took of my lifer Long-eared Owl. I guess I will have to develop another nemesis bird to keep myself challenged.

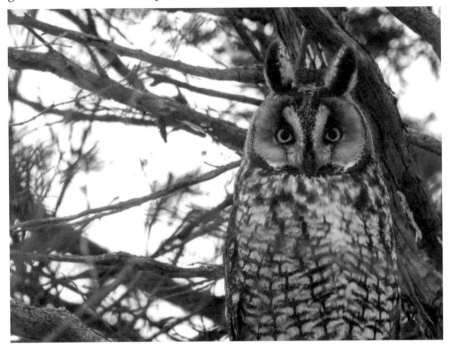

My ex-nemesis bird, the Long-eared Owl

One amusing challenge common to many birders is having such a strong desire to see a particular bird that one starts seeing things and imagines birds that are not there. Anticipation plus imagination can get the best of us, and often does! This is a common enough occurrence that there is actually a term for it, which I have heard frequently: *leaf bird*! I'm not going to provide excuses, such as poor light or pure exhaustion. Many times, I've become very excited about seeing a target bird sitting out in the open at the end of a branch, only to discover with my binoculars that it is actually an unusually shaped or positioned leaf, hence the expression. My mind has simply wished and willed that leaf into being what I want it to be. Errant leaves aren't the only pranksters to deceive birders; tent caterpillar nests are culprits as well. And then there are white plastic grocery bags: you only have to go looking for Snowy Owls once to learn how prolific plastic grocery bag litter is, even in remote, rural farm fields. Many times, I have stopped my car quickly when I was sure I'd spotted a distant Snowy Owl in a farmer's field, only to discover that it was actually a grocery bag.

And now, on a technically more serious note, I wish to touch on the scientific challenges of birding. In many species of birds, appearances vary by gender, age, and season. Males and females often look totally different; one extreme example is the Black-throated Blue Warbler, as shown in the following two photos. The female is so dissimilar to the male that early ornithologists thought she was an entirely separate species. The females of most species are much duller; their camouflage allows them to sit on a nest and raise a family (hopefully) undetected by predators. The difference in plumage between males and females is called sexual dimorphism. For whatever reason, in some species such as the Black-capped Chickadee, the Blue Jay, and the Canada Goose, there is no difference or only very subtle, minor differences between the sexes. A lack of sexual dimorphism seems to be more prevalent in species in which both parents tend to the nest and young.

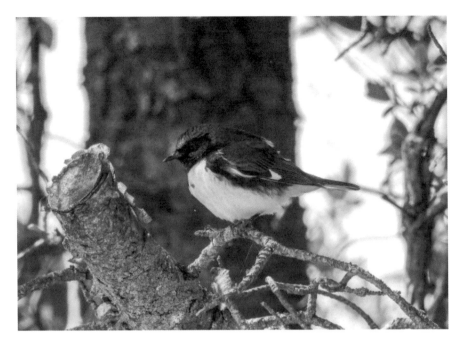

Male Black-throated Blue Warbler

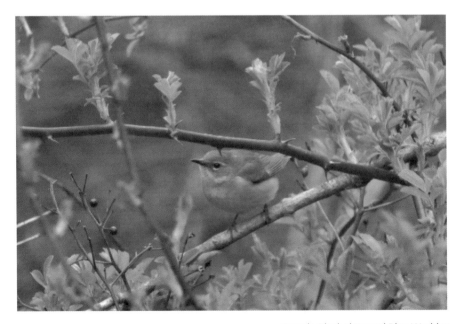

Female Black-throated Blue Warbler

In many species, the males, having bedazzled the females and successfully mated, lose their spring–summer breeding plumage and change into a much drabber, non-breeding plumage. It takes a lot of energy to produce flashy feathers, and their bright colours attract predators. An Audubon article titled *"Learn the Fall and Winter Colors of These Common Bird Species"* hilariously summarizes these changes this way: *"Birds in spring are dressed to kill, while birds in fall are dressed to chill. ... Like a fancy tuxedo on prom night or a few sessions in the tanning bed, many male birds put on their nicest duds each spring to impress. Once breeding season is over, though, it's back to sweatpants and stained T-shirts."*

To further confuse a novice birder, first-year hatch birds, both males and females, tend to look like their mothers, again, to provide extra camouflage until they grow up and are less vulnerable to predators. Hence, you might come across a description of a bird as a "female-type." This simply means the observer isn't sure if it is an adult female, a non-breeding male, or a juvenile of either sex.

The bottom line is that any given species might have three or four different "looks." These additional challenges add to the fun of birding. "Confusing fall warblers" is a common term, as many of the most colourful males in the spring morph into boring, bland birds in the fall. The result is that a few warbler species that you would never mistake in the spring when dressed in their dating finest end up all looking alike in the fall. Two of the best warbler examples of this are the Bay-breasted and Blackpoll Warblers. The males look entirely different in the spring and would never be confused with each other. However, come fall, they converge to the point that the main field mark to differentiate them is that the Blackpoll Warbler has yellow feet whereas the Bay-breasted's are dark. Some refer to these birds as "Baypolls," using a portmanteau to match their merged appearances.

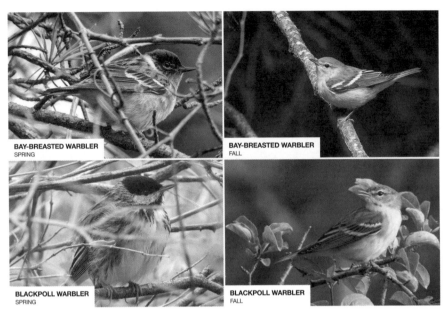

Comparison of Bay-breasted and Blackpoll Warblers, in breeding and non-breeding plumages

Another birding challenge is to learn their songs. I've met a number of birders who can identify hundreds of different species by sound alone, yet every bird usually has several songs, and to me they all are variations on a theme. I often get tricked when someone reports an exciting bird at some location and I go looking, only to realize they didn't actually see it, only heard it. To me, that doesn't count!

Finally, one other challenge is to have to deal with the aftermath of an inconsiderate birder, although thankfully this is rare. The vast majority of birders that I know are pleasant, respectful, and just plain wonderful people. There are always, of course, a few bad apples. Trespassing on private property to chase a bird can set off some landowners to the point where they become overtly hostile to everyone. I've even heard of landowners so aggrieved that they won't tolerate birders on public roads looking onto their property with binoculars.

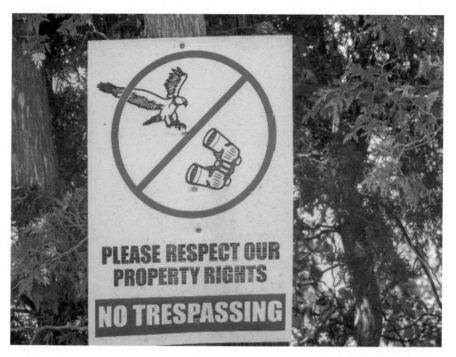

Are you looking at me?

This reminds me of a cartoon I once saw, showing two birds on a nest. One, looking quite angry, questions the other: "Are you watching the neighbors?" His response, while looking through binoculars, is, "It's a legitimate hobby!"

The bottom line is that we must always be respectful and not do something that could ruin it for everyone.

12. CATS!

To quote Monty Python, "And now for something completely different." You cannot love birds without talking about their nemesis, cats. Cats are to birds what Lyme-bearing ticks are to birders—a constant threat. My girlfriend Irina has always been cat-crazy but didn't want to have one while living in a high-rise in Toronto, having heard too many stories of cats escaping onto the balcony and then falling to their death or sustaining a crippling injury. I had never been a cat fan, as I found them so snotty and aloof. But my gratitude for having Irina in my life superseded my cat opinion, and that first Christmas together in 2015, my present was an "IOU one cat." It took a long time, surprisingly long to me, before Irina acted upon this. Later she admitted she had anxiety about getting a cat, knowing my animosity towards them.

But then we got Loshi, a Russian Blue. I don't know if it is characteristic of this breed to be so friendly and loving, or if it is just Loshi's wonderful personality. He comes to me to play, or to sleep on my lap; he is the perfect companion. If the doorbell rings, he is the first to the door to greet our visitor. To me he's got the best a dog has to offer, but without the barking or need to go out for a walk in the pouring rain or a blizzard for exercise or to do his business. I probably should have/could have written a book on how the perfect cat can help your Lyme symptoms. Loshi is love personified.

Like me, Loshi spends many hours watching birds through our windows. One day, however, he seemed a bit overwhelmed and nervous, when a flock of thirteen Wild Turkeys showed up. He wasn't used to seeing birds considerably larger than himself!

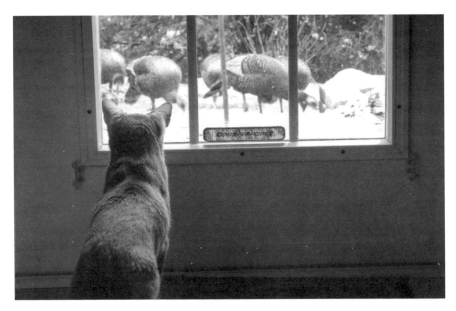

They're bigger than me! Loshi mesmerized by Wild Turkeys

If you look closely at the next photo, you will see Loshi is wearing a collar and is on a leash. If you love birds as much as I do, please, please, please do not let your cat roam free.

A 2013 study published by Environment Canada scientists concluded that free-roaming pet cats and feral cats are the number one killer of birds in Canada. The death toll is estimated at almost 200 million birds in Canada each year (and about 2.4 billion in the USA); collisions with power lines and buildings are a distant second, at about 51 million birds per year. I do not blame the cats; they are only doing what comes natural, as hunting is an instinctive action. It is the owners who are at fault. I have met a few who proclaim in all seriousness "But my Fluffy would never do that!" Right, want to bet? It's the same attitude that I encounter virtually every day when birding on park trails—dog owners letting their dogs run off-leash, ignoring the large, posted signs requiring them to be on leash at all times. I find there are a lot of dog owners who feel they and their pet are above the law. Dogs, typically rambunctious when running free, disturb and stress not only birds but mammals such as squirrels, chipmunks, and deer. I digress; this rant is about cats.

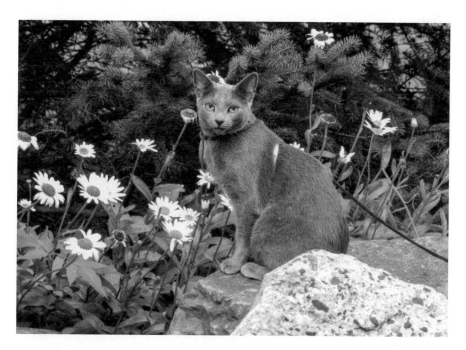

Loshi on a leash

I had a discussion once with a friend who argued, "It's just nature, cats killing birds." Yes, it *is* natural for the cats, however, it is *not* for our birds. Cats are not native to North America; they were brought on boats by early settlers to protect their provisions, required for their long trans-Atlantic journey, from stowaway mice and rats. Our birds did not evolve to be wary of cats stalking them.

Supposedly the average life span of an outdoor cat is two to five years, compared to fourteen for an indoor cat. I've discussed the fact that a few nestcams have revealed raptors bringing cats to their nestlings to eat. A recent study in the United States by the National Park Service found that twenty percent of urban coyotes' diets is made up of cats. Choosing to keep your cat indoors is not only safer for the birds, it is also safer for the well-being of your pet. Nature Canada runs an informative website called Cats and Birds where you can read up on what you can do to help protect both birds and cats.

Cat owners, your beloved pet should be chilling out in the window like Loshi, not out stalking and killing animals. Even adorable Loshi would do so if given the chance.

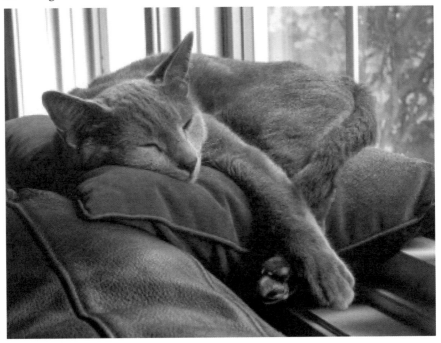

Proper hangout for your pet cat; Loshi resting in the window

13. LYME VALIDATION

Hopefully I've made my point that birding has been remarkable in helping me cope with Lyme disease and the chronic pains that come with it. Maybe I've even gained a few converts who are now considering birding as a coping mechanism for whatever ails them.

I have also tried to stress how frustrating it is to deal with the dismissive attitude towards Lyme disease, particularly chronic Lyme, that is prevalent throughout our conventional medical system. After a couple of fulfilling years of birding, I was quite happy to be done with fighting the medical establishment. However, since my Lyme diagnosis was primarily based on my symptoms, along with the IGeneX lab results, which only detect the body's response to the bacterial infections, not the actual bacteria, I was always on the lookout for different or new methodologies that could prove beyond a doubt that I have Lyme. I desired an indisputable diagnosis not because I wanted to win an "I told you so" argument with the doctors who had frustrated me. Rather, it was solely for my personal satisfaction: to have definitive proof that I was not crazy, and that I had not given up a career I loved at a financially inopportune time because of something that was all in my head.

A friend mentioned that there was a place not too far from my home that offers live blood microscopy. The health practitioner makes a couple of slides with smears of blood taken from a finger pinprick and displays them on a computer screen at high magnification. This practitioner could then visually identify various bacteria or parasites. I thought it would be fun to go and see what she might come up with.

I was "economic with the truth" in filling out the new patient form. I did not mention Lyme nor give a specific reason for why I was there; I simply said I was curious to see what I might be harbouring.

She started to move the slide slowly around on the microscope stage. It was neat to see my blood cells bobbing around, but even I could see the odd occasional white blob in between. She looked at me and asked if I scarfed down my food. I literally laughed out loud, as it is a common family tendency and I've been criticized my entire life for eating too fast. She said that the white blobs were the remnants of partially digested food that had leaked into my blood stream. When she correctly predicted my eating habits, I thought to myself, *this lady knows her business!* She then continued looking around the slide, when suddenly she squealed "Ooh, oh-oh!" I asked why she was so excited, and she said, "Oh, nothing, I need to keep looking." A minute later she got excited again, then looked at me and asked if I'd been exposed to a tick. I replied (truthfully), not that I was aware of, and she continued her study, and within a minute or two, again went "ooh," and said, "Are you sure you weren't exposed to a tick?" I then 'fessed up that I had Lyme, though I was not ever aware of a tick bite, and she said, pointing at the screen, "well, that's Babesia." I previously mentioned that the parasite Babesia is a co-infection with Lyme, and Dr. McShane had diagnosed me as having it. As she continued to move the slide around under the microscope lens, she spotted two additional Babesia cells.

After I had confessed that I have Lyme disease, she explained that she had been reluctant to tell me, as she didn't know if I was aware that I had it and therefore wasn't sure if she should be the one breaking the news to me that I had Lyme. We had both been playing a bit of a game. This was the first direct, in-your-face, positive evidence that I had seen which showed that I had a bacterial infection associated with Lyme. It may sound weird to be pleased with such a result, but it was gratifying to know that I wasn't crazy, that the IGeneX diagnosis was correct, and that Dr. McShane was as well. Furthermore, I had been right to be appalled by the dismissive, arrogant attitude from our conventional medical system that I'd encountered repeatedly. On a subsequent visit, she claimed that she spotted the Lyme spirochete. She took screen-capture images and made mini-videos of my blood's activity.

I am living with Lyme disease and I have seen indisputable, photographic proof. I could now go back to birding, content with the knowledge that this new passion was helping me to cope with a physical disease that I definitely did have.

14. THE RIFE MACHINE AS THERAPY

In January 2018, I attended a dinner and ceremony for Terry MacGibbon, the founder and chairman of the board of the company where I served as CEO, when he was inducted into the Mining Hall of Fame. Yes, that's a real thing: there is a Canadian Mining Hall of Fame. It was my first interaction with former colleagues and friends since my retirement in the fall of 2015. One of the company's board members told me that subsequent to my retirement, his wife had contracted Lyme and been cured using a Rife machine. He said that I was welcome to borrow it. Being a scientist, I was highly skeptical of this technology, which I will explain briefly, but as someone living with chronic pain, I was willing to try anything. I would never have gone down this path if I hadn't been offered the use of the machine, as they cost roughly $5,000 (Canadian).

The history and efficacy of the Rife machine is steeped in mythology and conspiracy theories. I am not going to delve into a detailed history or description, but will provide a summary. Interested readers can do their own research and reach their own conclusions. Katina Makris gives an excellent review in her book *"Out of the Woods, Healing from Lyme Disease for Body, Mind, and Spirit."*

The Rife technology was developed in the 1920s and 1930s by Dr. Royal Raymond Rife, a scientist-physician, working in a lab in California. Initially Rife invented a new optical microscope that purportedly exceeded the powers of all other technology of the day; it was capable of viewing, for the first time, living pathogenic organisms such as bacteria and viruses. Conventionally, such organisms were dead when being examined. Rife went on to postulate that bacteria and viruses all have an electromagnetic vibration; they resonate at a unique frequency. Rife referred to this frequency as the mortal oscillatory rate (MOR). He invented and designed the Rife machine to duplicate MOR frequencies and inundate the body with the ones that matched whatever particular bacterial or viral infection was present. His theory was that, by subjecting the body to electromagnetic radiation at the appropriate frequency, the disease-causing microorganism would resonate so strongly that it would be disabled or killed, analogous to an opera singer who can vocalize at the right frequency to break a wine glass. Although Rife did not state he could cure cancer, he did believe his technology could "devitalize" the organisms causing it.

Rife is reported, at least according to the mythology surrounding him, to have been successful in treating many forms of cancer as well as other diseases such as typhus. This breakthrough was so respected that in 1931 a group of America's top medical authorities met to honor Rife, with then Southern California American Medical Association (AMA) president Dr. Millbank Johnson declaring "The End to All Disease." Unfortunately for Rife, at about the same time, the pharmaceutical industry was rapidly ascending in size and political power. Recently developed wonder-drugs included penicillin and cortisone; there was a push for doctors to prescribe drugs and a push against anything that might reduce potential profits.

The AMA even went so far to hire someone to track down any alternative medical treatments that they did not support. The Rife machine was obviously a potential threat to the pharmaceutical industry. This is where the story becomes mysterious and akin to conspiracy theories. I refer the reader to an article by Barry Lynes, called *The Cure for Cancer and AIDS May Already Exist*.

In a nutshell, Rife was apparently harassed out of work and died penniless and embittered that the conventional medical system had conspired to reject his findings. Or, did the system successfully put someone running a health fraud out of business? I have no idea and am not qualified to comment nor recommend. I can only speak for my own experience, and as I said, the reader needs to research and reach their own conclusions.

Frequency generator machines of various types have been revived by the complementary medicine field to treat a number of illnesses, including Lyme. These devices have been the subject of a number of health fraud cases and have not been certified or approved by either the American or Canadian governments.

This brings me back to the conversation that I chanced to have with my former colleague, the company director who offered the use of his Rife machine. He advised that all I had to do was go to Michigan to see a complementary practitioner who specialized in the Rife machine. She would run a comprehensive scan on me, to determine a list of the various infections

I had, based on their MOR frequencies. With that list, she could then write a computer program that cycled through the various frequencies the Rife would pulse through my body to target and kill whatever specific bacteria or viruses I harbored. The concept was similar to the galvanic skin test I had earlier, which had originally determined that I have Lyme.

Off I went to Ann Arbor, Michigan, and was told by the Rife practitioner that I had ten different strains of the Lyme bacteria along with four co-infections. She claimed that most Lyme patients have up to thirty strains, and the fact that I was down to ten was probably due to the previous antibiotic treatments I'd been on. I was given a program to run thirty times, every other day for two months. The program would take two hours and seven minutes to cycle through the various frequencies being pulsed into me.

I returned home and contacted my former colleague to determine how to get his machine. He seemed a bit vague and, after a week or so, he admitted his wife was still using it, but not to worry—he'd figure it out. Several days later, there was a FedEx delivery man at my front door with a parcel for me. My colleague had bought me a brand-new machine! I was brought to tears, a combination of gratitude and my Lyme-ravaged emotions. I'll never forget his kind words: "I just want to see you better, buddy."

The Rife machine I was given is used in conjunction with a saline footbath containing a device that has two metal plates with a low-level current arcing between them. Supposedly the dead Lyme bacteria and toxins are secreted through the pores of your skin and into the footbath, if you are using this particular model of machine. In an entertaining Canadian Broadcasting Corporation documentary (Doc Zone) Bob McDonald travels to an anti-aging symposium in Las Vegas and deftly debunks numerous examples of fraudulent "snake oil." He tries a footbath connected to a frequency generator machine (not a Rife machine), and the water turns brown and gunky; like my Rife machine this is supposedly due to the dead material excreted through the skin of the feet. He then runs a foot bath without his feet in it, and the water still turns brown and gunky. McDonald points out that the discolouration and material are actually due to rapid oxidation of the metal plates. In spite of this skepticism, I was now in possession of a brand new, $5,000 Rife machine and had just spent over $600 to have the scan and resulting program to run, so therefore was willing to proceed.

I finished my thirtieth treatment around Christmas 2018 and went back to see the Rife practitioner in Michigan in January 2019. I was feeling highly skeptical as she scanned me, since I didn't feel any improvement. I was astounded to hear her saying how good things were looking. I was down to six strains of Lyme, from ten, and had only one co-infection, down from four. She wrote a new, shorter program, of just over one hour, and recommended twenty treatments, done every other day. The shorter program was because there were fewer frequencies required to be run due to the reduced number of targeted bacteria. At the end of those sessions I once again made the pilgrimage to Ann Arbor, still not feeling any better, and this time the scan revealed that all of my co-infections were gone, but that I had six "new" strains of Lyme. This seemed rather suspicious to me, as if it were just to keep me coming back for additional treatments, but I was assured that this is not uncommon—the new strains were Lyme bacteria that had been "hiding out" inside various parasites and co-infection bacteria. When those died off, the Lyme bacteria were liberated and thus became detectable. I was given one final new program to run for a couple of months. Over those two months I noticed that suddenly the severity of all of my symptoms diminished, and for the first time in several years, I felt reasonably good. Upon completion of this third round of treatment, I returned to Ann Arbor, where her scan showed no evidence of any Lyme or co-infections in me. She was quick to say that it didn't mean that my symptoms would be completely gone; some would take months if not years to disappear, as my body repaired and recovered from the damage already inflicted. Some symptoms such as neurological issues might never disappear, due to permanent damage caused by the now-defeated bacteria.

Although I remain skeptical of the science behind the Rife machine, it certainly did something to ease my pains, fatigue, and neuropathy. In the spring of 2019, I participated in a week-long birding trip in Mexico organized by Barry Coombs. The days were all long, with typical 5:30 a.m. departures, and we would return around 4 or 5 p.m., at which point most of the other participants would rest, whereas I'd walk to a local park and continue birding until dark, which was around 7 p.m. Such long days were a far cry from previously needing a daily afternoon nap.

One of our birding locations was on a trail with nearly a thousand-foot total change in elevation—and this started at 8,200 feet above sea level. I knew I was doing much better when I handled this as well as any of the other participants. Before starting the Rife treatment, I could not have climbed such hills at home in southern Ontario, never mind at high altitude. Pre-Rife, I would become winded and my legs would turn to mush simply climbing the stairs in my house.

Since that trip to Mexico, my fatigue has increased a bit, such that I go through periodic cycles of needing a daily nap, and my neuropathy, crepitus, and tinnitus are worse again. However, overall, I am much better and now riding my stationary bike up to sixty minutes a day. The Rife treatment certainly seems to have helped me. That does not mean it will work for everyone, and all I can recommend is that anyone interested conduct their own investigations and research prior to committing to such a large financial expenditure.

15. BIRDING AS THERAPY

For me, birding's effectiveness as therapy is related to its status as a form of meditation or "mindfulness." It gets you to focus on the moment and to block out all extraneous thoughts, worries, anxieties, and noise that our brains are so great at churning up. People pay good money to participate in mindfulness courses, workshops and retreats. Courses and group learning can be great. However, whether as an adjunct or an alternative to them, just step out into nature, and listen to and watch birds going about their lives. You don't have to be as obsessive as I am about birds, or purchase expensive cameras and binoculars. Simply watch, listen, and learn from the birds; they are providing the best therapy I can find for free. When birding, whether from my window, sitting in my backyard, walking a trail, or wherever it may be, I feel calm, at peace, and am oblivious to my pains. Nothing makes me happier or more content than birding: seeing and hearing birds singing, establishing territory, finding a mate, protecting a nest, and raising and feeding their young.

It is not just the birds that are therapeutic. To me, there is nothing like walking in fresh air and communing with nature to feel content and relaxed, allowing me to forget that my body hurts. Watching clouds race by the sun, hearing the wind rustling in the leaves or the sounds of a babbling brook, hearing and seeing bees buzzing and butterflies flitting about—all of these are soothing and therapeutic, good not only for the mind and soul but the body as well. I even find that food tastes better when eaten outdoors; a snack or lunch while out birding tastes fantastic. The famous neurologist and author Dr. Oliver Sacks wrote, in an essay on gardens, that in his professional experience there were only two types of non-pharmaceutical "therapy" that were beneficial for patients with chronic neurological diseases: music and botanical gardens. Sacks stated, "*I cannot say exactly how nature exerts its calming and organizing effects on our brains, but I have seen in my patients the restorative and healing powers of nature and gardens, even for those who are deeply disabled neurologically. In many cases, gardens and nature are more powerful than any medication.*" I would add that a key element of the soothing experience of spending time in a botanical garden is the presence of its birds, and that consciously listening to and watching birds going about their lives will only enhance the restorative and healing powers of the experience.

Birding is not necessarily just a casual hobby or a science; as I've discussed in the politics of birding, for many, it's often treated as a competitive sport. It is almost a state of mind more than anything. It is like a pro athlete "getting in the zone," locked in, totally focused, such that nothing can distract. I was out birding with friends and, unbeknownst to me, Bill McDonald took the photo of me in Chapter 8. You can see that I'm in the zone, oblivious to being photographed.

I'm not alone in finding birding therapeutic. For several years, Joe Harkness from England wrote a blog called *Bird Therapy* that focused on how birding helps with mental health, including stress, anxiety and depression. The blog, now defunct, led to Mr. Harkness successfully crowd-funding a book, *Bird Therapy*, which was published in the summer of 2019.

There is a blog called *Anxious Birding* written by Ian Young, in which he discusses the mental health benefits of birding. In his May 30, 2017, blog he writes: *"In my mind, I want to be far away from here, in a vast wilderness. There will be no one else around and I will be overwhelmed by natural beauty. The constant noise of real life will be replaced by the splashing of a river, the howling of the wind and the cries of wild creatures."* Sure sounds idyllic and soothing to me!

In an interesting article in *Psychology Today*, titled *"The Power of Nature: Ecotherapy and Awakening"*, author Steve Taylor states, *"In recent years, researchers have become aware of a powerful new kind of therapy, which is just as effective against depression as traditional psychotherapy or medication. And the amazing thing is that you don't have to pay for this therapy. It's free, and completely accessible to anyone at any time. It's not even a new therapy either—in fact, it's even older than the human race. This is ecotherapy—contact with nature. A few years ago researchers at the University of Essex in 2007 found that, of a group of people suffering from depression, ninety percent felt a higher level of self-esteem after a walk through a country park, and almost three-quarters felt less depressed. Another survey by the same research team found that ninety-four percent of people with mental illnesses believed that contact with nature put them in a more positive mood. Since then, in the UK, contact with nature has been increasingly used as a therapy by mental health professionals."*

I came across an article on the *Good News Network* called *"Watching Birds Near Your Home is Good For Your Mental Health,"* which references a University of Exeter survey that found that there are mental health benefits to being able to see birds and trees, bushes, and shrubs, regardless of whether you live in a lush, leafy suburb or a more urban environment. Furthermore, it points out that the particular species of birds made no difference; more important was the number of birds that can be seen, from your windows or in your yard or neighbourhood. For me, the more birds the better, but having become a dedicated birder, the individual species *is* very important to me. Don't get me wrong, seeing the same birds over and over never gets boring, but seeing a rare bird or one new to me gives me a bigger "high" and therefore does an even better job of taking my mind off my body.

Famous birders Kenn and Kimberly Kaufman provide an excellent summary of the benefits of birding in an article they wrote for *Birds and Blooms* titled *"Birding For Your Health: Discover how birdwatching can do wonders for your physical and mental well-being."* Another article well-worth reading, by Greg Presto, is titled *"Birdwatching Is an Easy Way to Practice Mindfulness."* A woman in England, Francesca Baker, learned to deal with her anorexia by sitting by the window and watching birds. Like me, she took pride in learning to identify various species and then over time built up the energy to go for drives to see more birds.

As you can see, I can take no credit for discovering the benefits of birding and being out in nature. The articles referenced above focus on the mental health benefits, whereas I've found that birding provides physical benefits as well. Those physical benefits aren't, of course, permanent and are related to my state of mind; but they certainly put my physical pains into a state of suspended animation when my brain is focused on the excitement of birding. To me, the word *birds* is an acronym for "birding inevitably reduces disease symptoms!"

16. EPILOGUE

It is appropriate that I began to write this book in 2018, which was proclaimed the Year of the Bird, and finished it in 2021, while the world remains in the grip of the novel coronavirus COVID-19 pandemic.

In 1918, the Migratory Bird Treaty Act was enacted by Canada and the United States. It has served as the strongest bird protection law ever passed. It makes it illegal to take or possess, import or export, transport, buy, sell, or barter any migratory bird, including their parts, nests or eggs, unless under the terms of a government permit issued pursuant to the regulations. One hundred years ago, there was a large trade in birds and bird feathers, which were in fashion, mostly for fancy hats. This demand led to steep declines in Snowy Egret and other beautiful shorebirds. A boycott against feather use in fashion led to the eventual formation of the Audubon Society and directly to the Migratory Bird Act.

To honour the centennial of the act, the Cornell Lab of Ornithology, the National Audubon Society, National Geographic, and BirdLife International teamed up with millions of people worldwide as well as more than one hundred other conservation organizations to celebrate 2018 as the Year of the Bird. As a result, there was a lot more press about birds, birding, and bird therapy.

What does the current pandemic have to do with birding? People confined to their local neighbourhoods or homes all over the world began to discover the therapeutic benefits of birding, and of nature in general. I have described previously how avid birders will carry out a "Big Year" in which they try to achieve a record number of species sightings, and how this was the theme of the entertaining movie *The Big Year*. The Cornell Lab of Ornithology sponsors a Global Big Day, held annually in early May. During the May 9, 2020, event, 50,000 participants submitted to eBird a single-day record of 120,000 checklists, comprising 2.1 million bird observations of 6,479 species. This was thirty percent more checklists than the previous record, resulting in more information being uploaded to eBird in one day than during its first two and half years in existence. These statistics reflect a trend that has been occurring since the pandemic started to isolate and quarantine people in March 2020. With their usual choices of entertainment suddenly unavailable, people began to discover the joys of birding from wherever they could access, whether "socially distanced" in local parks, or from their own windows and balconies at home. Many found it comforting and reassuring to see birds continuing the business of their daily lives, while the routines of their own daily lives were so drastically altered. In a May 27, 2020 blog, the American Bird Conservancy gave testimonials from ten individuals on how "How Birds Inspired Us During A Pandemic: 10 Stories Of Cheer (& Chirps)."

In late 2019, my friend Carter Dorscht, who as I previously mentioned runs an Algoma District birding Facebook group, organized and launched an Ontario-wide challenge for 2020 called 5MR, the MR standing for *mile radius*. The challenge is for a birder to find as many species as possible within a five-mile radius circle centred on his or her home. Above and beyond the friendly, competitive nature of the challenge are two purposes: first, to help build databases in under-birded areas, and second, to help reduce a birder's carbon footprint caused by chasing rare birds and frequently traveling to birding hotspots far from home. Little did Carter know that he could not have chosen a better year to run this challenge! With many beloved birding hot spots such as Point Pelee closed during spring migration, thanks to COVID-19 restrictions, birders couldn't stray far from home anyway. For me personally, it has been an eye-opening exercise, having discovered a diverse number of excellent bird habitats (more habitats equal more birds) and therefore excellent birding spots that I did not know existed so close to home. I was thrilled to end the year having seen 175 species within my five-mile radius circle. This has given me great comfort to realize that, as I get older and perhaps develop additional health issues (whether they are Lyme-related or not) which might prevent me from traveling far from home, I will still be able to get "my fix" of satisfying birding without suffering from birding FOMO.

The outbreak of the pandemic is another reminder of our need to take better care of our home planet, which is suffering so much abuse at our hands. There is considerable anecdotal evidence that birds were doing just fine without us when our lives were shut down by the pandemic. Birds are the "canary in the coal mine" when it comes to climate change, habitat loss, and other environmental considerations; they are excellent indicators of the integrity of ecosystems and environmental health. These beautiful creatures symbolize the interconnectivity of nature and the importance of taking better care of our one and only planet. For example, a study published in 2019 revealed that in North America, over the past fifty years our bird population has declined by almost thirty percent, for a net loss of 2.9 billion birds. Birds that inhabit grasslands, such as the Eastern Meadowlark and Bobolink, suffered the greatest decline of fifty-three percent, a loss of more than 700 million individual birds. This is likely primarily due to habitat loss as a result of the use of more toxic pesticides, agricultural intensification, and development.

Climate change is probably a key driver in the rapid expansion of Lyme disease, allowing ticks to expand their range northwards and forcing birds that inadvertently carry and spread ticks to modify and adapt their breeding ranges as well. In fact, a young woman from Vancouver Island in British Columbia is currently suing the Canadian federal government to compel it to develop a climate change action plan, because she claims the Lyme disease she contracted is due to climate change expanding the habitat of disease-transmitting ticks.

I have many birding friends whose attitude about contracting Lyme range from uptight to downright paranoid. After all, as birders we want to be chick magnets, not tick magnets! I am obviously no expert when it comes to avoiding Lyme, however I firmly believe that you must not let your fear or anxiety of contracting Lyme ruin your hobby and passion. In my opinion, the benefits of what you are doing outweigh the risks. The most effective way to avoid struggling with Lyme disease is to prevent contracting it. As long as you take sensible precautions such as staying on the trails and out of tall grasses, tucking your pants into your socks, and doing a thorough body check for ticks afterwards, the odds are with you. You can search online for a recipe to make your own natural tick-repellant spray. On the website *Instructables Living,* a fellow named Matt Makes provides some tips on how to avoid tick bites, what to do if you do suffer one, how to remove an embedded tick, and an interesting recipe for tick spray made with neem, citrus, and garlic.

Just remember that not every "bug" bite is a tick bite, that not every tick is a Black-legged Tick, and that not every Black-legged Tick is carrying Lyme.

I find nothing more calming and spiritual than being out in nature. The ethereal, timeless sound of wind blowing in the pine trees takes me to my happy place; a bird in the pine tree is a bonus. When we're physically active outdoors and breathing fresh air, we tend to take longer, slower, deeper breaths. The additional oxygen makes us more alert and puts us in a better mood, and the time in the sun boosts our vitamin D levels, which helps to alleviate anxiety and depression, and fight infection.

Lyme totally changed my life. It forced me to retire from an exciting, challenging, well-paying job that I loved. Lyme is what, indirectly, led me to birding, and while I wouldn't wish Lyme on anyone, I am grateful to have ended up as a happy birder, even with my physical limitations, or more to the point, my "lyme-itations." Birding saved my life. It brings me excitement, fun, new challenges, peace of mind, satisfaction, and most importantly, takes my mind off my body.

Irina pointed out that I have totally reinvented myself. I am now living in a new home, with a new partner, with a pet that I adore (even though my entire life I have disliked cats), I have made an entirely new set of friends (not to say I've discarded the old ones!), and I have a new science discipline, having essentially traded geology for ornithology. For over thirty-five years as a geologist, the acronym BIF meant to me "banded iron formation"; now, in my new birder lingo, it refers to "birds in flight."

Irina's comment about reinventing myself led me to some soul-searching introspection. Lyme has indeed changed my life, but it isn't all for the worse. Yes, it has been years since I could remember what it felt like to be totally pain-free. Yes, my finances were impacted by having to retire prematurely. But on the other hand, I am no longer living on an airplane and out of a suitcase, constantly worn out and stressed. While working, I never really appreciated how stressed I was; I had been running on adrenalin without realizing it. But now my biggest daily decision is whether to go birding or not, and if so, where. I realize that I have found inner peace and happiness.

The tired old cliché "When life gives you lemons, make lemonade" is actually an excellent proverb for how to live your life. Always look on the bright side of life, as the Monty Python group sang in their movie *Life of Brian*. While my father lay dying from pancreatic cancer, he would often say, "I'm just taking it one day at a time."

I think that the most important thing to help deal with a chronic illness, not just Lyme, is to throw yourself into something that you are passionate about: something you can focus on, derive pleasure from, and that gets your mind off the lousy hand you've been dealt health-wise. Of course, it depends on your level of physical ability. Riding a horse may be totally soothing and calming for some, but if that is too physically demanding, perhaps spending time in a horse stable will do just as well, or even watching videos of horses from bed. Perhaps it is quilting, or sewing, or reading, or binging on Netflix. It is not important what it is; what is important is that it helps you, soothes you, and provides you a new focus and passion in life that, even temporarily, gets your mind off of being sick.

Life is a journey, and it is incumbent on us to make the best of it. I hope my journey might inspire some folks suffering with a chronic illness to get out of the "Lyme light" and into the sunlight, where the singing birds will warm your heart and lift your spirits.

17. ACKNOWLEDGMENTS

Two people in particular deserve a shout-out for the prominent roles they played in inspiring and encouraging me to write this book. I owe a huge thank-you to my niece Emily Kerton, of Thunder Bay, Ontario, for originally proposing the concept. Emily, who runs outreach programs in northwestern Ontario for Sudbury, Ontario–based Science North, shares my nature interests, and we have gone birding together several times. It was in 2018, while we were birding in the Sax-Zim Bog in Minnesota, that she proposed the idea. I would never have thought of it without her inspiration. After Emily's suggestion, I wrote a bit but then moved on to other things and of course continued to spend most of my time birding. In the meantime, this project went dormant. To borrow a baseball analogy, if Emily was the starter, then Jeanne Lise Pacey, who runs the Hamilton (Ontario) Regional Lyme Alliance, was the closer. After I had the pleasure of meeting Jeanne and happened to mention that I'd started this, she encouraged me to keep going and finish it, and provided a number of valuable insights. Jeanne's Facebook page for her Hamilton group contains a wealth of valuable information on Lyme disease that she frequently updates. So, thanks to you both, Emily and Jeanne!

Along the frustrating path that Lyme has taken me, two very supportive friends played key roles in guiding me towards a proper diagnosis. First, my good friend Sara Kernan, who, fairly soon after my mysterious symptoms began, suggested that I might have Lyme disease. Amongst all my acquaintances, Sara was unique in having a friend with Lyme disease, so she had first-hand familiarity with it. Sara recognized that my symptoms were similar to those of her friend Pierrette Donaghy. Not only did this plant the seed in my head that I might have contracted Lyme, I gained a new friend in Pierrette, who I could commiserate with and relate to. Pierrette and I communicated by email or phone calls for several years before we finally met face to face in March 2019—a classic Lyme patient scenario of one or both of us being too ill to get together. Pierrette continues to be not only a wonderful friend but also a great source of numerous articles and links to informative stories on Lyme.

The second friend who was instrumental in me getting a diagnosis is Jamile Cruz, a business colleague who recommended I be tested by a complementary health practitioner who had correctly diagnosed an ailment she had. This practitioner was the first to state that I had Lyme, thus confirming Sara's prescient hunch.

In the birding world, I have made many new friends; three, in particular, have mentored me and, at the risk of a bad pun, taken me under their wings. I extend my gratitude to my friends Bill McDonald of Kitchener, Ontario; Barry Coombs of Hamilton, Ontario; and Peter Thoem of Burlington, Ontario. They have all been generous with their time and knowledge, and graciously put up with numerous, undoubtedly annoying questions. The sheer joy, fun, comfort and relaxation that birding provides me, and my camaraderie with these gentlemen, has led me to say, only half-jokingly, that Lyme disease was the best thing that ever happened to me!

Finally, I would be remiss if I did not mention Dr. Irina Kuslya. We began dating prior to me contracting Lyme, and Irina has stood by me and supported me, above and beyond what anyone could ever ask. I don't think I would be in a position to write this book if not for her steadfast, loving support.

I must stress that I am a geologist, not a medical doctor. Although I've now lived with Lyme for almost nine years and have read several text books on it as well as numerous papers and articles, I am not an expert. I can only relate my own understanding and experience. I hope this book will encourage those suffering with chronic pain to take up binoculars or a camera and experience birding therapy. Simply writing about what I've experienced has been cathartic for me.

Finally, this book has benefited from some excellent editing and suggestions by several dear friends and relatives. In particular I thank Ed O'Connor, a birding friend who just happens to be a professional editor, and my daughter Candace, whose suggestions were uncannily similar to Ed's. I am responsible for any errors or omissions that remain.

18. NOTES

When my favourite band: In the early 1970's Robert Plant would introduce Stairway to Heaven with the comment "this is a song of hope"; this is memorialized on Led Zeppelin's live album "The Song Remains the Same." I saw Led Zeppelin perform at Pontiac Silverdome in Michigan on April 30, 1977. The concert, with 77,229 in attendance, set a world record for the largest audience for a single-act performance: https://www.ledzeppelin. com/show/april-30-1977. To have been in such a large indoor crowd seems surreal after living for more than a year with severe restrictions, closures, and stay-at-home orders as a result of the pandemic.

Alex Trebek, the long-time host: A simple internet search will lead you to numerous quotes from this beloved TV game show host; for example: https://quotefancy.com/alex-trebek-quotes. I chose to highlight this particular quote, not just for the fact that I am in total agreement with it, but also for who said it. Trebek was from Sudbury, Ontario, where my children were born and where I began my career as a geologist with Inco Limited.

Chapter 1
Page 11
It is important to point out that I did not look sick: This (usually) well-intentioned saying, that can be easily taken the wrong way, is just one of many statements that can be upsetting to those suffering from a chronic illness. In a December 1, 2018 article entitled "18 Common 'Pet Peeves' of People with Chronic Illness", Paige Wyant compiled a list of such annoyances: https://themighty.com/2018/12/chronic-illness-common-frustrations-pet-peeves/.

Chapter 4
Page 29
The Global Lyme Alliance states that the ELISA test is falsely negative nearly 50% of the time: This frustrating fact is provided on their website https://globallymealliance.org/about-lyme/diagnosis/testing/.

Page 30
To quote Yogi Berra, this was "déjà vu all over again": The famous baseball
player is probably more famous, or infamous, for his never-ending
malapropisms. Probably the two best known are "It ain't over 'til it's
over" and "It's deja vu all over again": https://www.today.com/news/
its-deja-vu-all-over-again-27-yogi-berras-most-t45781.

Page 30
However, Lyme can also present a smorgasbord of seemingly unrelated,
strange symptoms: I recommend an article from *The Atlantic* "Lyme Disease
Is Baffling, Even to Experts", written by Meghan O'Rourke, a Lyme patient:
https://www.theatlantic.com/magazine/archive/2019/09/life-with-lyme/594736/.

Page 32
Ontario veterinarians treat dogs for Lyme disease: Like all things tick-related,
there are inconsistencies amongst Canadian veterinarians in their level of
tick knowledge, prevention, and care. However, this paper makes clear that
our dogs appear to get better medical care than their owners, including
screening and vaccinations: "Assessing knowledge, attitudes, and practices
of Canadian veterinarians with regard to Lyme disease in dogs": https://doi.
org/10.1111/jvim.16022.

Page 35
I find it intriguing that Canada's provincial and federal governments,
and medical community: This reference is from the first of a five-part
series on MS by Dani-Elle Dubé of Global News, published on May 14,
2018: "Brain Interrupted, Multiple sclerosis in Canada: Understanding
why MS rates are the highest here": https://globalnews.ca/news/4191203/
multiple-sclerosis-canada-understanding-why-ms-rates-are-the-highest-here/.

Page 35
In December 2018, the Toronto Star published an excellent article: Although
frustrating in the extreme, I found this article by Isabel Teotonio, entitled
"Lyme disease is steeped in controversy. Now some doctors are too afraid to
treat patients", published on December 14, 2018, to be weirdly comforting;

to know my experience with the medical community was not unique and that many others unfortunately have gone through the same challenges as I have: https://www.thestar.com/life/health_wellness/2018/12/14/everything-about-lyme-disease-is-steeped-in-controversy-now-some-doctors-are-too-afraid-to-treat-patients.html.

Chapter 5

Page 50

In addition, the topography leads to the city of Hamilton's claim: The Niagara Escarpment runs through Hamilton, which is situated at the west end of Lake Ontario. The "mountain", as locals call it, provides dramatic scenery and vistas overlooking the lake, and thanks to the topography, there are about 130 waterfalls within the city limits. Cassie Shortsleeve wrote an informative story "Why Hamilton, Canada is the Waterfall Capital of the World", for Condé Nast Traveler, published on July 24, 2017: https://www.cntraveler.com/story/why-hamilton-canada-is-the-waterfall-capital-of-the-world.

Page 52

Scrambling to prepare for the meeting: Cornell's website has always been my go-to source of information on birds, and it didn't disappoint. I found a 2009 research paper titled "External characteristics of houses prone to woodpecker damage." Written by Emily G. Harding, Sandra L. Vehrencamp, and Paul D. Curtis, it can be found at https://digitalcommons.unl.edu/cgi/viewcontent.cgi?article=1030&context=hwi.

Page 53

My talks even got promoted in a local newspaper: I presume the Hamilton library system put this ad in the local paper: "Backyard Birds of Hamilton, ON May 25, 2017": https://www.hamiltonnews.com/events/7216960--backyard-birds-of-hamilton/.

Page 56

CBD is an extract from the cannabis plant: When searching for any health-related information on the internet, I will only use reputable sites, given how many questionable "web doctors" will pop up in a search. My preferred

site is the Mayo Clinic; you can read more about CBD oil here: https://
www.mayoclinic.org/healthy-lifestyle/consumer-health/expert-answers/
is-cbd-safe-and-effective/faq-20446700.

Chapter 7
Page 59
Considering that at any given time there are between 200 billion and
400 billion individual birds in the world: I found this interesting tidbit
on the American Museum of Natural History's website: https://www.
amnh.org/explore/ology/earth/ask-a-scientist-about-our-environment/
how-big-is-the-bird-population.

Page 59
According to Birds Canada, twenty-five percent of Canadian households
have bird feeders: Bird seed and products is a big business. Even where I
live, there are a couple of huge sunflower farms within a half-hour drive of
home. Mark and Ben Cullen reviewed the benefits to the birds of us feeding
them, and provided the statistics, in a February 11, 2017 article in The Toronto
Star: "Birds' survival deserves a boost beyond bird feeders": https://www.
thestar.com/life/homes/2017/02/11/birds-survival-deserves-a-boost-beyond-
bird-feeders.html. More detailed statistical data can be found in a study
called "Canadians and Nature: Birds, 2013" on Statistics Canada's website
at https://www150.statcan.gc.ca/n1/pub/16-508-x/16-508-x2015001-eng.htm.

Page 69
The current understanding of the reason for a Snowy Owl irruption is actually
counterintuitive: Project SNOWstorm provides a wealth of information on
Snowy Owls. You can read up on irruptions on their website: https://www.
projectsnowstorm.org/what-is-an-irruption/.

Page 76
Evolution is very creative at providing different strategies for reproduction:
Brown-headed Cowbirds have been known to parasitize the nests of more
than 220 species of birds. You can read more about them on Cornell's Lab

of Ornithology website "All About Birds": https://www.allaboutbirds.org/ guide/Brown-headed_Cowbird/overview.

Page 78

One interesting webcam is based at the top of the Sheraton Hotel: The Hamilton Community Peregrine Project began in 1994 when someone observed a Peregrine Falcon hanging around the rooftop of the Sheraton Hotel in downtown Hamilton. Careful monitoring efforts began in 1995 after it became apparent there was a nesting pair on the ledge of the eighteenth floor of the hotel. Details of this project along with links to video feed can be found at falcons.hamiltonnature.org.

Page 78

For example, there is a feedercam in Manitouwadge, in northwestern Ontario: This feedercam is run by Tammie Haché as part of Cornell's Project FeederWatch. It is of particular interest to me as the feeders attract many boreal bird species including Pine and Evening Grosbeaks, Common Redpolls, Canada Jays, and even Ruffed Grouse. There have also been some interesting vagrants such as a Western Meadowlark. To view the feedercam go to https:// www.allaboutbirds.org/cams/ontario-feederwatch/. Tammie Haché wrote an article entitled "Virtual birding north of Lake Superior" which was published in OFO News, Newsletter of the Ontario Field Ornithologists, Volume 36, Number 3, October 2018.

Page 78

There is a website called Bird Feeder Webcams: This site, which can be found at https://www.viewbirds.com/feeders.htm, provides links to cameras at feeders, watering holes and stations, and migration stopover sites, in over thirty countries. In addition, it provides a link to another site which lists various cameras on bird nests.

Chapter 8

Page 79

Over my first winter of retirement: The very active Hamilton Naturalists' Club is over 100 years old, growing out of the Hamilton Bird Protection

Society founded in 1919. There are over 600 members, including many with expertise on the local flora and fauna, not just birds. To see all that it offers, visit https://hamiltonnature.org/.

Page 82
There is also a similar Ontario-wide: The Ontario rare bird alert listserv is administered by the Ontario Federation of Ornithologists. It, along with several other alerts available by email, Discord, or Facebook, can be accessed at http://www.ofo.ca/site/content/ontario-hotlines-and-news.

Page 84
Any decent bookstore, or store that specializes in bird feeding, such as Wild Birds Unlimited, will have a good selection to choose from: Wild Birds Unlimited is my go-to store for all things bird related. I'm lucky to have two outlets within a reasonable distance of my home, one in Burlington, and one in Guelph.

Page 85
In an article titled "The best birding apps are ones tied to bird guidebooks," Jim Williams: In this informative article, published in the Star Tribune on December 4, 2018, Jim Williams provides a brief overview of a number of birding apps, including several I use, such as iBird Pro, Merlin Bird ID, and The Warbler Guide. This article can be accessed at https://www.startribune. com/the-best-birding-apps-are-ones-tied-to-bird-guidebooks/501895072/.

Page 86
Cornell's Lab of Ornithology has a free app you can download called Merlin Bird ID: Merlin is the must have birding app, especially for beginners. You can read all about it on their website at http://merlin.allaboutbirds.org/ help-and-faqs/, and there is a link on that page to download it for free.

Page 86
It typically gives two or three choices, especially for very similar species: In the spring/summer 2017 issue of Caltech magazine Robert Perkins wrote a brief review of Merlin which can be found at https://magazine.caltech.edu/ post/merlin-bird-photo-id. Merlin was launched in 2014 and is continuously

improving as the database behind it grows in leaps and bounds thanks to eBird contributors.

Page 86
Their All About Birds website is my go-to resource: It will be apparent that the Cornell Lab of Ornithology is my favourite source of information. You can find it at https://www.allaboutbirds.org.

Page 87
Take the Wood Thrush: The traditional range map found in any field guide or bird reference book is a fixed map like the Wood Thrush example that I provided. I obtained it from Wikimedia, with attribution to Cephas, CC BY-SA 4.0 <https://creativecommons.org/licenses/by-sa/4.0>, via Wikimedia Commons.

Page 87
Compare that map to the new abundance maps eBird can produce: Thanks to the hundreds of millions of contributions of citizen scientists to their eBird database, Cornell Lab of Ornithology can now produce range maps that are more like intensity maps, such that one can see where the frequency of a species is more common within its overall range. This Wood Thrush abundance map was taken from https://ebird.org/science/status-and-trends/ woothr/abundance-map. It provides far more information on the distribution of Wood Thrush than the old-fashioned traditional range map. Full accreditation for this map can be found in References under Fink et al.

Page 89
For those interested in knowing more about eBird: This introductory course to eBird can be accessed via https://academy.allaboutbirds.org/product/ ebird-essentials/.

Page 89
In addition to Cornell, there are numerous other excellent bird websites: The Audubon Guide to North American Birds can be accessed at https:// www.audubon.org/bird-guide, while the Boreal Songbird Initiative's

Comprehensive Guide to Boreal Birds is at https://www.borealbirds.org/comprehensive-boreal-bird-guide.

Page 92
I suggest you refer to an article titled "Birding Blind: Open Your Ears to the Amazing World of Bird Sounds" by Trevor Attenberg: This is a heartwarming story of a legally blind young man who found solace, joy, and a connection to nature by learning to bird by ear. His story was published on Audubon's website on October 18, 2018: https://www.audubon.org/news/birding-blind-open-your-ears-amazing-world-bird-sounds.

Page 93
Birders are a strange lot: Yes, we are! Science writer, nature cartoonist, and naturalist Rosemary Mosco wrote all about birding in cemeteries for Audubon on October 5, 2018: "The Ins and Outs of Birding With the Dead": https://www.audubon.org/news/the-ins-and-outs-birding-dead.

Page 94
If you are up to traveling to a new spot: Birding Pal is a brilliant concept, connecting travelers interested in birding with local birders. The first thing that caught my eye when I visited the Birding Pal website, at http://www.birdingpal.org/, was the option to view it in dozens of different languages, which demonstrates just how broad its international reach is, and how global interest in birding is. Anyone on a quick business trip or vacation with a few hours to spare might be able to squeeze in some quality birding by utilizing this site.

Chapter 9
Page 95
Birders love to keep lists: Matthew Miller, wrote "Birding for People Who Do Not Like Lists" for Cool Green Science on April 10, 2108. In the article, he comments how he is "struck by their mania for organization and lists", referring to birders planning trips to maximize sightings, plotting big days and big years with the efficiency of military campaigns, and logging sightings

on spreadsheets and apps: https://blog.nature.org/science/2018/04/10/
birding-for-people-who-do-not-like-lists/.

Page 96
Perhaps it was inevitable in this digital era: For armchair birders or those
grounded by inclement weather, one can sign up to participate in Fantasy
Birding on their webpage at https://fantasybirding.com/.

Page 97
I admit, though, that if there is a bird: Missing out on a rarity which has
been seen by all of your friends can be crippling. Purbita Saha even wrote an
article on this for Audubon, published on May 18, 2018: "How to Deal With
Birding FOMO": https://www.audubon.org/news/how-deal-birding-fomo.

Page 98
On January 11, 2019, a European Robin showed up on the grounds of the
Beijing Zoo: The word "twitching" might be a British term for chasing rare
birds, but it is clearly a universal passion amongst birders. The huge throng
of birders with their impressive array of cameras shown in the photo on
the blog Birding Beijing could have been taken anywhere in the world
where birding is a common hobby: https://birdingbeijing.com/2019/01/11/
brexit-refugee-european-robin-given-warm-reception-in-beijing/.

Chapter 10
Page 116
On September 22, 2019, Tina Survilla Lindell, quoting a birder whom she
had met, tweeted: "There's no cure. Birdwatching is terminal. When you get
it, you got it for life." Ms. Lindell tweets under the handle @ParallelLindell.

Chapter 11
Page 121
An Audubon article titled "Learn the Fall and Winter Colors of These
Common Bird Species." This article, authored by Nicholas Lund,
was published on Audubon's website on September 28, 2018. I abso-
lutely love his colourful description of the difference in male bird's

breeding and non-breeding plumages: https://www.audubon.org/news/
learn-fall-and-winter-colors-these-common-bird-species.

Chapter 12
Page 126
A 2013 study published by Environment Canada scientists: One of my
biggest pet peeves is the fact that so many millions of birds are unnecessarily
slaughtered every year by pet and feral cats. The source for this disgusting
fact is a paper published in the Avian Conservation & Ecology journal, which
can be found at http://www.ace-eco.org/vol8/iss2/art11/. The full reference to
this interesting science paper is: Calvert, A.M., C.A. Bishop, R.D. Elliot, E.A.
Krebs, T.M. Kydd, C.S. Machtans, and G.J. Robertson, 2013. A synthesis of
human-related avian mortality in Canada. Avian Conservation and Ecology
8(2): 11. http://dx.doi.org/10.5751/ACE-00581-080211.

Page 127
A recent study in the United States by the National Park Service found
that twenty percent of urban coyotes' diets is made up of cats: If the threat
that your beloved, free-roaming cat might meet its demise as a coyote's
dinner doesn't convince you to obey the law and keep your cat indoors,
nothing will. Katherine Gammon wrote an article entitled "High-cat diet:
urban coyotes feast on pets, study finds", published in The Guardian on
February 12, 2019: https://www.theguardian.com/environment/2019/apr/12/
protect-your-pets-cats-make-up-one-fifth-of-coyotes-diet-in-los-angeles.

Page 127
Nature Canada runs an informative website: Well-worth visiting this site
to better inform yourself on this topic near and dear to my heart: https://
catsandbirds.ca/.

Chapter 14
Page 131
The Rife technology was developed in the 1920's and 1930's by Dr. Royal
Raymond Rife: There is so much controversy and mythology associated
with the Rife machine and its purported efficacy that I encourage anyone

suffering from Lyme and considering it as a treatment to carefully do their own research before expending large sums of money. It certainly seemed to be the turning point in my recovery but I remain skeptical enough that I'm not prepared to recommend it. I've derived the information on it from several sources, including Wikipedia (https://en.wikipedia.org/wiki/Royal_Rife), an excellent book by Katina Makris on her journey with Lyme, called "Out of the Woods, Healing from Lyme Disease for Body, Mind, and Spirit", "The Royal R. Rife report", by Alison Davidson, and a November 1987 article by Barry Lynes, titled "The Cure for Cancer and AIDS may already exist", published in the Consumer Health Newsletter Vol. 9, Number 10.

Page 133
In an entertaining Canadian Broadcasting Corporation documentary (Doc Zone): Anyone interested in Rife-type technology will find this forty-four-minute-long documentary worth watching: https://www.dailymotion.com/video/x50084v.

Chapter 15
This chapter includes numerous references to articles that describe the mental health benefits of both birding and nature in general. My experience has been that birds aren't only good for the mind and soul, but for the physical body as well. Birds enthrall me to the point that my mind forgets that it is connected to an aching body, and I believe that this level of focused engagement with the natural world, birding or otherwise, can do the same for others with chronic pain as well.

Page 137
Sacks stated, "I cannot say exactly how nature exerts its calming and organizing effects on our brains, but I have seen in my patients the restorative and healing powers of nature and gardens, even for those who are deeply disabled neurologically. In many cases, gardens and nature are more powerful than any medication." I found it very gratifying to have such a preeminent world expert concur with my own views. This quote is from a New York Times article called "The Healing Power of Gardens", published on April 18, 2019. The article is an excerpt from a posthumous collection of writings

by Dr. Sacks titled "Everything in its Place." The New York Times article can be found at: https://www.nytimes.com/2019/04/18/opinion/sunday/oliver-sacks-gardens.html.

Page 138
There is a blog called Anxious Birding: This blog about birding and mental health, by Ian Young, can be found at https://anxiousbirding.wordpress.com/.

Page 138
In an interesting article in Psychology Today, titled "The Power of Nature: Ecotherapy and Awakening": This article, by Steve Taylor, was posted on Psychology Today's website on April 28, 2012: https://www.psychologytoday.com/ca/blog/out-the-darkness/201204/the-power-nature-ecotherapy-and-awakening.

Page 139
I came across an article on the Good News Network called "Watching Birds Near Your Home is Good For Your Mental Health": This story, which I can totally relate to, can be found at https://www.goodnewsnetwork.org/watching-birds-near-home-good-mental-health/.

Page 139
Famous birders Kenn and Kimberly Kaufman provide an excellent summary: Pay attention to any article with either of these two listed as an author. They are not only informative and very knowledgeable, but also have a gift and flair for writing. This particular story, titled "Birding for your Health: Discover how birdwatching can do wonders for your physical and mental well-being", was originally published in Birds & Blooms on December 15, 2013 and given a pandemic update on May 12, 2020: http://www.birdsandblooms.com/birding/birding-basics/birding-health/.

Page 139
Another article well-worth reading, by Greg Presto: Presto's article, titled "Birdwatching is an Easy Way to Practice Mindfulness", was published on Vice's website on March 18, 2020: https://tonic.vice.com/en_us/article/evq457/birdwatching-mindfulness-meditation-benefits-birding.

Page 139

A woman in England: In "Watching my Way to Wellness" Francesca Baker tells a heartwarming story of how birding helped her recover from anorexia; it was published on the Folks website: https://folks.pillpack.com/watching-my-way-to-wellness/.

Chapter 16

Page 141

It is appropriate that I began to write this book in 2018, as 2018 was proclaimed the Year of the Bird: You can read more about the Year of the Bird in an article written by Rhiannon L. Crain, entitled "2018 Is the Year of the Bird. See 3 Ways to Celebrate at Home", published on Houzz: https://www.houzz.com/ideabooks/104455584/list/2018-is-the-year-of-the-bird-see-3-ways-to-celebrate-at-home.

Page 141

In 1918, the Migratory Bird Treaty Act was enacted by Canada and the United States: Wikipedia provides a wonderful amount of detail on this far-sighted, brilliant legislation: https://en.wikipedia.org/wiki/Migratory_Bird_Treaty_Act_of_1918.

Page 141

During the May 9, 2020 event: This is from a Cornell Lab of Ornithology press release titled "Birdwatchers Set World Records On Global Big Day", issued on May 15, 2020 and published at https://mailchi.mp/cornell/news-release-birdwatchers-break-records-on-global-big-day-1317584.

Page 142

In a May 27, 2020, blog, the American Bird Conservancy gave testimonials: The American Bird Conservancy published on their website "How Birds Inspired Us During A Pandemic: 10 Stories Of Cheer (& Chirps)." This is a very timely collection of anecdotes illustrating how so many people were touched by birds and benefited from bird watching as a solace during the pandemic lockdowns: https://abcbirds.org/blog20/birds-during-pandemic.

Page 142
There is considerable anecdotal evidence that birds were doing just fine without us: In a May 29, 2020 New York Times opinion piece titled "What Birds Do for Us and What We Can Do for Them", author Jennifer Ackerman describes how, during the pandemic, people have been more aware of the birds around them, and how the birds seem to have been enjoying the quieter, shuttered world: https://www.nytimes.com/2020/05/29/opinion/sunday/coronavirus-lockdowns-birds-nature.html. In Appendix B, Resources, one of the bird books I recommend is Ackerman's "The Genius of Birds."

Page 143
For example, a study published in 2019 revealed that in North America: In a paper titled "Decline of the North American Avifauna", written by Rosenberg, Kenneth V. et al and published October 4, 2019 in Science, the authors present shocking data: there has been a net loss approaching three billion birds: https://science.sciencemag.org/content/366/6461/120.full.

Page 143
In fact, a young woman from Vancouver Island in British Columbia is currently suing the Canadian federal government: A Canadian Press reporter, Amy Smart, wrote the article "Youths file lawsuit over climate inaction" in the October 25, 2019 National Post: https://nationalpost.com/pmn/news-pmn/canada-news-pmn/youths-file-lawsuit-with-federal-court-calling-ottawa-to-develop-climate-plan/.

Page 143
On the website Instructables Living: Matt Makes wrote a highly informative article on tick prevention, titled "Natural Tick Repellent and Tips for Keeping Ticks Away": https://www.instructables.com/id/Natural-Tick-Repellent-and-Tips-for-Keeping-Ticks-/. In it he provides a recipe and instructions on how to make a natural tick repellent, other measures you can take to avoid a tick bite, and, if all else fails, how to remove an embedded tick.

19. REFERENCES

Ackerman, Jennifer, May 29, 2020: What Birds Do for Us and What We Can Do for Them, in *The New York Times* https://www.nytimes.com/2020/05/29/opinion/sunday/coronavirus-lockdowns-birds-nature.html

American Bird Conservancy, May 27, 2020: How Birds Inspired Us During A Pandemic: 10 Stories Of Cheer (& Chirps) https://abcbirds.org/blog20/birds-during-pandemic

American Museum of Natural History: https://www.amnh.org/explore/ology/earth/ask-a-scientist-about-our-environment/how-big-is-the-bird-population

Attenberg, Trevor, 2018: Birding Blind: Open Your Ears to the Amazing World of Bird Sound; https://www.audubon.org/news/birding-blind-open-your-ears-amazing-world-bird-sounds

Baker, Francesca: Watching my Way to Wellness https://folks.pillpack.com/watching-my-way-to-wellness/

Bauer, Brent A.: What are the benefits of CBD-and is it safe to use? *Mayo Clinic* https://www.mayoclinic.org/healthy-lifestyle/consumer-health/expert-answers/is-cbd-safe-and-effective/faq-20446700

Bird Feeder Webcams: https://www.viewbirds.com/feeders.htm

Birding Beijing: https://birdingbeijing.com/2019/01/11/brexit-refugee-european-robin-given-warm-reception-in-beijing/

Calvert, A.M., C.A. Bishop, R.D. Elliot, E.A. Krebs, T.M. Kydd, C.S. Machtans, and G.J. Robertson, 2013: A synthesis of human-related avian mortality in Canada. *Avian Conservation and Ecology* 8(2): 11. http://dx.doi.org/10.5751/ACE-00581-080211

Canadians and Nature: Birds, 2013: *Statistics Canada* https://www150.statcan.gc.ca/n1/pub/16-508-x/16-508-x2015001-eng.htm

Cats and Birds: http://catsandbirds.ca/

Cephas-Evans, M., E. Gow, R.R. Roth, M.S. Johnson, and T.J. Underwood (2011) Wood Thrush (Hylocichla mustelina), version 2.0. In *The Birds of North America* (A. F. Poole, Editor). Cornell Lab of Ornithology, Ithaca, NY, USA. https://doi-org.acces.bibl.ulaval.ca/10.2173/bna.246, CC BY-SA 4.0 https://commons.wikimedia.org/w/index.php?curid=69056339taken

Chillag, Amy, November 13, 2018: Birdwatching for peace of mind and better health https://www.cnn.com/2018/11/12/health/sw-birding-for-health/index.html

Clifton, Mark, August 12, 2019: The beginner's guide to the greatest pastimes: Birding *CBC Life* https://www.cbc.ca/life/culture/the-beginner-s-guide-to-the-greatest-pastimes-birding-1.5244307

Cornell Lab of Ornithology: All About Birds https://www.allaboutbirds.org

Cornell Lab of Ornithology: Brown-headed Cowbird https://www.allabout-birds.org/guide/Brown-headed_Cowbird/overview

Cornell Lab of Ornithology, May 15, 2020: Birdwatchers Set World Records On Global Big Day: https://mailchi.mp/cornell/news-release-birdwatchers-break-records-on-global-big-day-1317584

Crain, Rhiannon L., February 23, 2018: 2018 Is the Year of the Bird. See 3 Ways to Celebrate at Home https://www.houzz.com/ideabooks/104455584/list/2018-is-the-year-of-the-bird-see-3-ways-to-celebrate-at-home

Cullen, Mark and Ben, *The Toronto Star*, February 11, 2017: Birds' survival deserves a boost beyond bird feeders https://www.thestar.com/life/homes/2017/02/11/birds-survival-deserves-a-boost-beyond-bird-feeders.html

Curry, Robert, 2006: Birds of Hamilton and Surrounding Areas

Davidson, Alison, date unknown: The Royal R. Rife report, published by Borderland Sciences

Doc Zone (CBC), 2014: Magical Mystery Cures with Bob McDonald https://www.dailymotion.com/video/x50084v

Dubé, Dani-Elle, May 14, 2018: Brain Interrupted, Multiple sclerosis in Canada: Understanding why MS rates are the highest here https://globalnews.ca/news/4191203/multiple-sclerosis-canada-understanding-why-ms-rates-are-the-highest-here/

Dunne, Pete, 2006: Pete Dunne's Essential Field Guide Companion

Earley, Chris G., 2012: Hawks & Owls of Eastern North America

Earley, Chris G., 2003: Sparrows & Finches of the Great Lakes Region & Eastern North America

Earley, Chris G., 2003: Warblers of the Great Lakes Region & Eastern North America

Earley, Chris G., 2005: Waterfowl of Eastern North America

Fantasy Birding: https://fantasybirding.com/

Fink, D., T. Auer, A. Johnston, M. Strimas-Mackey, O. Robinson, S. Ligocki, W. Hochachka, L. Jaromczyk, C. Wood, I. Davies, M. Iliff, L. Seitz. 2021. eBird Status and Trends, Data Version: 2020; Released: 2021. Cornell Lab of Ornithology, Ithaca, New York. https://doi.org/10.2173/ebirdst.2020

Frank, Anne, 1952: The Diary of a Young Girl

Gammon, Katharine, April 12, 2019: High-cat diet: urban coyotes feast on pets, study finds https://www.theguardian.com/environment/2019/apr/12/protect-your-pets-cats-make-up-one-fifth-of-coyotes-diet-in-los-angeles

Global Lyme Alliance: https://globallymealliance.org/about-lyme/diagnosis/testing/

Good New Network, 2018: Watching Birds Near Your Home is Good For Your Mental Health https://www.goodnewsnetwork.org/watching-birds-near-home-good-mental-health/

Haché, Tammie 2018: Virtual birding north of Lake Superior in *OFO News*, Newsletter of the Ontario Field Ornithologists, Volume 36, Number 3, October 2018

Hamilton Community Peregrine Project: falcons.hamiltonnature.org

Hamilton News, May 25, 2017: Backyard Birds of Hamilton https://www.hamiltonnews.com/events/7216960--backyard-birds-of-hamilton/

Hamilton Regional Lyme Alliance: https://www.facebook.com/groups/438944952893144/

Harding, Emily G., Vehrencamp, Sandra L., and Curtis, Paul D. Spring 2009: External characteristics of houses prone to woodpecker damage https://digitalcommons.unl.edu/cgi/viewcontent.cgi?article

Harkness, Joe, 2019: Bird Therapy

Kaufman, Kenn and Kimberly, May 12, 2020: Birding for your Health: Discover how birdwatching can do wonders for your physical and mental well-being http://www.birdsandblooms.com/birding/birding-basics/birding-health/

Led Zeppelin, 1976: Movie "The Song Remains the Same"

Led Zeppelin: https://www.ledzeppelin.com/show/april-30-1977

Lund, Nicholas, September 28, 2018: Learn the Fall and Winter Colors of These Common Bird Species https://www.audubon.org/news/learn-fall-and-winter-colors-these-common-bird-species

Lynes, Barry, November 1987: The Cure for Cancer and AIDS May already exist *Consumer Health Newsletter* Vol. 9, Number 10

Makes, Matt Natural Tick Repellent and Tips for Keeping Ticks Away: https://www.instructables.com/id/Natural-Tick-Repellent-and-Tips-for-Keeping-Ticks-/

Makris, Katina I., 2015: Out of the Woods, Healing from Lyme Disease for Body, Mind, and Spirit

Merlin Bird ID: https://merlin.allaboutbirds.org/help-and-faqs/

Migratory Bird Treaty Act: https://en.wikipedia.org/wiki/Migratory_Bird_Treaty_Act_of_1918

Miller, Matthew L., April 10, 2018: Birding for People Who Do Not Like Lists https://blog.nature.org/science/2018/04/10/birding-for-people-who-do-not-like-lists/

Mosco, Rosemary, October 5, 2018: The Ins and Outs of Birding With the Dead https://www.audubon.org/news/the-ins-and-outs-birding-dead

Moss, Stephen, May 4, 2019: Natural high: why birdsong is the best antidote to our stressful lives *The Guardian* https://www.theguardian.com/environment/2019/may/04/birdsong-antidote-to-stressful-lives-dawn-chorus-day

Nichol, Grace K., Weese, J. Scott, Evason, Michelle, and Clow, Katie M., January 9, 2021: Assessing knowledge, attitudes, and practices of Canadian veterinarians with regard to Lyme disease in dogs: in *Journal of Veterinary Internal Medicine*, Volume 35, Issue 1: https://doi.org/10.1111/jvim.16022

O'Rourke, Meghan, September 2019: Lyme Disease is Baffling, Even to Experts *The Atlantic* https://www.theatlantic.com/magazine/archive/2019/09/life-with-lyme/594736/

Perkins, Robert, 2017: Merlin Bird ID, in *Caltech magazine*, spring/summer 2017: https://magazine.caltech.edu/post/merlin-bird-photo-id

Pittaway, Ron: Winter Finch Forecast 2018-2019, http://jeaniron.ca/2018/wff18.htm

Pope, Richard, 2009: The Reluctant Twitcher: A Quite Truthful Account of My Big Birding Year

Presto, Greg, March 18, 2020: Birdwatching Is an Easy Way to Practice Mindfulness https://tonic.vice.com/en_us/article/evq457/birdwatching-mindfulness-meditation-benefits-birding

Project SNOWstorm: https://www.projectsnowstorm.org/what-is-an-irruption/

Rosenberg, Kenneth V. et al, October 4, 2019: *Science* Vol. 366, Issue 6461: Decline of the North American Avifauna: https://science.sciencemag.org/content/366/6461/120.full

Rousseau, Steve, April 11, 2017: You Should Get into Birding, the Most Relaxing of Hobbies http://digg.com/2017/how-to-go-birding

Sacks, Dr. Oliver, April 18, 2019: The Healing Power of Gardens *The New York Times* https://www.nytimes.com/2019/04/18/opinion/sunday/oliver-sacks-gardens.html

Saha, Purbita, May 18, 2018: How to Deal With Birding FOMO https://www.audubon.org/news/how-deal-birding-fomo

Shortsleeve, Cassie, July 24, 2017: in *Condé Nast Traveler* https://www.cntraveler.com/story/why-hamilton-canada-is-the-waterfall-capital-of-the-world

Smart, Amy, October 25, 2019: Youths file lawsuit over climate inaction *National Post* https://nationalpost.com/pmn/news-pmn/canada-news-pmn/youths-file-lawsuit-with-federal-court-calling-ottawa-to-develop-climate-plan/

Stephenson, Tom and Whittle, Scott, 2013: The Warbler Guide

Stump, Scott, September 23, 2015: 'It's deja vu all over again': 27 of Yogi Berra's most memorable 'Yogi-isms' in Today https://www.today.com/news/its-deja-vu-all-over-again-27-yogi-berras-most-t45781

Taylor, Steve, 2012: The Power of Nature: Ecotherapy and Awakening, *Psychology Today* https://www.psychologytoday.com/ca/blog/out-the-darkness/201204/the-power-nature-ecotherapy-and-awakening

Teotonio, Isabel, December 14, 2018: Lyme disease is steeped in controversy. Now some doctors are too afraid to treat patients in *The Toronto Star* https://www.thestar.com/life/health_wellness/2018/12/14/everything-about-lyme-disease-is-steeped-in-controversy-now-some-doctors-are-too-afraid-to-treat-patients.html

The Big Bang Theory: CBS sitcom 2007-2019

Thorne-Ithology: A Boy's-eye View of Birding https://thorne-ithology.
    blogspot.com/
Trebek, Alex: https://quotefancy.com/alex-trebek-quotes
Wikipedia: "Royal Rife" https://en.wikipedia.org/wiki/Royal_Rife
Williams, Jim, December 4, 2018: The best birding apps are
    ones tied to bird guidebooks http://www.startribune.com/
    the-best-birding-apps-are-ones-tied-to-bird-guidebooks/501895072/
Wyant, Paige, December 1, 2018: 18 Common 'Pet Peeves' of
    People with Chronic Illness https://themighty.com/2018/12/
    chronic-illness-common-frustrations-pet-peeves/
Young, Ian: Anxious Birding https://anxiousbirding.wordpress.com/

20. APPENDIX A: BIRD EXPRESSIONS

I introduced Chapter 7, Backyard Birding for Beginners, by stating that we use numerous bird-related expressions in our everyday conversations. This is a more exhaustive list of such idioms and expressions. I'm sure there are more that I didn't think of.

- A bird in the hand is worth two in the bush
- A chicken and egg situation
- An albatross around your neck
- As dead as a dodo
- As free as a bird
- As the crow flies
- Bird brain
- Birds of a feather flock together
- Birds-eye view
- Chicken out
- Chickens come home to roost
- Cold turkey
- Crazy as a loon
- Didn't mean to ruffle your feathers
- Don't count your chickens before they hatch
- Eagle eye
- Eat crow
- Feather in your cap
- Fly the coop
- Get your ducks in a row
- Goose bumps
- Great weather, if you're a duck
- Happy as a lark
- He/she's no spring chicken
- His goose is cooked
- Jail bird
- Kill the goose that laid the golden egg

- Kill two birds with one stone
- Lame duck
- Like a duck takes to water
- Like water off a duck's back
- Night owl
- Pecking order
- Proud as a peacock
- Run around like a chicken with his head cut off
- Sitting duck
- Spread one's wings
- Swan song
- Talk turkey
- The early bird catches the worm
- Ugly duckling
- Under their wings
- What's good for the goose is good for the gander
- Wild goose chase

21. APPENDIX B: RESOURCES

The following is a collection of all the Lyme- and birding-related resources suggested throughout the text. Many of the birding resources are southern Ontario specific, but not all. In addition, I've provided a brief commentary on a few books on birds and on Lyme that I enjoyed and recommend.

READING
Bird Guides and Books on Birding

- *Bird Therapy* – Joe Harkness
- *Birding without Borders* – Noah Strycker
- *Birds of Hamilton and Surrounding Areas* – Robert Curry
- *Hawks & Owls of Eastern North America* – Chris Earley
- *Pete Dunne's Essential Field Guide Companion* – Pete Dunne
- *Sparrows & Finches of the Great Lakes Region & Eastern North America* – Chris Earley
- *The Warbler Guide* – Tom Stephenson and Scott Whittle
- *Warblers of the Great Lakes Region & Eastern North* America – Chris Earley
- *Waterfowl of Eastern North America* – Chris Earley

Other Books on Birds That I Recommend

- *The Genius of Birds* – Jennifer Ackerman. This book will leave you with a newfound respect for the incredible intelligence exhibited by birds. Never again will you use the expression "bird brain" unless meaning it as a compliment.
- *The Hidden Lives of Owls* – Leigh Calvez. In my experience, even those most disconnected from and uninterested in nature still love owls and are fascinated by them; I mentioned that when I give bird presentations, I always leave the owls for last, for fear of peaking too soon. Leigh Calvez's book will only increase your admiration for these beautiful, mystical birds.

- *The Reluctant Twitcher: A Quite Truthful Account of My Big Birding Year* – Richard Pope. Along the line of Strycker's *Birding without Borders*, I found this book appealing, as the "twitching" was done in my neck of the woods, describing some places just a few kilometres from my house. *Twitching* is a British term for chasing rare birds.
- *What the Robin Knows* – Jon Young. This is one of the most informative bird books I've ever read. Young totally gets you into the head of various birds to understand what they are thinking when they exhibit certain behaviours. Through careful observation of bird behaviour you can open yourself up to understanding the dynamics of their daily struggle to thrive and survive.
- *What It's Like to Be a Bird* – David Allen Sibley. This famous birder/artist has produced an informative, entertaining book that is good for all ages.
- *Kingbird Highway* – Kenn Kaufman. Famous birder and author Kaufman chronicles his coming-of-age big year birding experiences in the 1970s; must reading for anyone interested in birding.

Articles on Birding for Mental Health (see Notes or References for links)

- *Birding Blind: Open Your Ears to the Amazing World of Bird Sounds* – Trevor Attenberg
- *Birding for your Health: Discover how birdwatching can do wonders for your physical and mental well-being* – Kenn and Kimberly Kaufman
- *Birdwatchers Set World Records On Global Big Day* – Cornell Lab of Ornithology
- *Birdwatching for peace of mind and better health* – Amy Chillag
- *Birdwatching is an Easy Way to Practice Mindfulness* – Greg Presto
- *How Birds Inspired Us During A Pandemic: 10 Stories Of Cheer (& Chirps)* – American Bird Conservancy
- *Natural high: why birdsong is the best antidote to our stressful lives* – Stephen Moss

- *The Healing Power of Gardens* – Dr. Oliver Sacks
- *The Power of Nature: Ecotherapy and Awakening* – Steve Taylor
- *Watching Birds Near Your Home is Good For Your Mental Health* – Good News Network
- *Watching my Way to Wellness* – Francesca Baker
- *What Birds Do for Us and What We Can Do for Them* – Jennifer Ackerman

General Articles on Birding (see Notes or References for links)

- *2018 Is the Year of the Bird. See 3 Ways to Celebrate at Home* – Rhiannon L. Crain
- *Birding for People Who Do Not Like Lists* – Matthew Miller
- *How to Deal With Birding FOMO* – Purbita Saha
- *The beginner's guide to the greatest pastimes: Birding* – Mark Clifton
- *The Ins and Outs of Birding With the Dead* – Rosemary Mosco
- *You Should Get into Birding, the Most Relaxing of Hobbies* – Steve Rousseau

Books on Lyme Disease

- *Why Can't I Get Better? Solving the Mystery of Lyme & Chronic Disease* – Dr. Richard Horowitz. Horowitz is one of the most renowned Lyme doctors in the United States. This book is heavy reading but well worth the effort if you want to better understand this disease and the challenges of treating it.
- *Ending Denial – The Lyme Disease Epidemic: A Canadian Public Health Disaster* – Helke Ferrie. This compilation is frustrating reading. That is not a criticism; it is frustrating as it brings back all the memories of futile dealings with the medical system and continually running into a brick wall. This book should be mandatory reading for all Canadian politicians and medical doctors.
- *Out of the Woods: Healing from Lyme Disease for Body, Mind, and Spirit* – Katina I. Makris with a foreword by Richard Horowitz.

For lighter reading, this is an excellent story of one individual's journey with Lyme. Following her memoir, which serves as part one of her book, Katina provides an in-depth, comprehensive overview of Lyme disease, including signs and symptoms, prevention, testing, and various treatment options.

Articles on Lyme Disease (see Notes or References for links)

- *Assessing knowledge, attitudes, and practices of Canadian veterinarians with regard to Lyme disease in dogs* – Nichol, Grace K. et al
- *Lyme Disease is Baffling, Even to Experts* – Meghan O'Rourke
- *Natural Tick Repellent and Tips for Keeping Ticks Away* – Matt Makes

DIGITAL MEDIA
Websites

- Andrew Mactavish's blog *Bird Snaps: Birding and Photography*: https://birdsnapsblog.blogspot.com/
- Audubon Guide to North American Birds: https://www.audubon.org/bird-guide
- Barry Coombs's blog *The Experienced Intermediate Birder*: www.experiencedintermediatebirder.wordpress.com
- Bill McDonald's blog *Grenfell's Nature Blog*: https://grenfell.weebly.com/
- Bill McDonald's photography website *TEKFX Photography*: http://tekfx.ca/
- Bird Feeder Webcams: https://www.viewbirds.com/feeders.htm
- Birdfilms: http://www.birdfilms.com/
- Birding Beijng: https://birdingbeijing.com/2019/01/11/brexit-refugee-european-robin-given-warm-reception-in-beijing/
- Birding Pal: http://www.birdingpal.org/
- Comprehensive Guide to Boreal Birds https://www.borealbirds.org/comprehensive-boreal-bird-guide
- Cornell's eBird: https://ebird.org/home
- Fantasy Birding: https://fantasybirding.com/

- Hamilton Community Peregrine Project: falcons.hamiltonnature.org
- Hamilton Naturalists' Club: https://hamiltonnature.org/
- Ian Young's blog *Anxious Birding*: https://anxiousbirding.wordpress.com/
- Ontario FeederWatch (Manitouwadge): https://www.allaboutbirds.org/cams/ontario-feederwatch/
- Ontario Field Ornithologists: http://www.ofo.ca/
- Peter Thoem's blog *My Bird of the Day*: http://www.mybirdoftheday.ca/
- Project SNOWstorm: https://www.projectsnowstorm.org/what-is-an-irruption/
- The Cornell Lab of Ornithology *All About Birds* website: https://www.allaboutbirds.org/
- Thorne-Ithology: A Boy's-eye View of Birding https://thorne-ithology.blogspot.com/

Facebook Groups/Pages

- Advanced Birding in Ontario: https://www.facebook.com/groups/1955395661363064/
- Algoma District Birding: https://www.facebook.com/groups/algomadistrictbirding/.
- Birds, Blooms, Beasts, Bugs and Butterflies: https://www.facebook.com/groups/1584723541822039/
- Doug Ward: https://www.facebook.com/doug.ward.948494
- Friends of Sam Smith Park: https://www.facebook.com/groups/969873946403806/
- Hamilton Region Lyme Alliance: https://www.facebook.com/groups/438944952893144/
- Ontario Bird Photography: https://www.facebook.com/groups/ontariobirdphotography
- Ontario Birds: https://www.facebook.com/groups/377736792291721/
- Ontario Owls: https://www.facebook.com/groups/1091175727561101/
- Ontario Rare Bird Alert: https://www.facebook.com/groups/376660149346593/

- Rondeau: https://www.facebook.com/groups/275384882852428/
- Sax-Zim Bog: https://www.facebook.com/groups/saxzimbog/

Flickr Pages

- Ed O'Connor: https://www.flickr.com/photos/152894743@N08/
- Randy Droniuk: https://www.flickr.com/photos/26679916@N03/
- Steve Rossi: https://www.flickr.com/photos/sspike

Twitter Accounts

- Jim Pottkotter: @HappyPixr
- Mali: @MaliHalls
- Maranda Mink: @Marandamink
- The Inept Birder: @TheIneptBirder

Videos and Online Courses

- Be a Better Birder: Duck and Waterfowl Identification, Cornell Lab of Ornithology
- Be a Better Birder: Hawk & Raptor Identification Archived Series, Cornell Lab of Ornithology
- eBird Essentials: https://academy.allaboutbirds.org/product/ebird-essentials/
- Magical Mystery Cures: https://www.dailymotion.com/video/x50084v
- Owl Power
- Spring Field Ornithology–Northeast, Cornell Lab of Ornithology
- The Big Year
- The Great Courses: The National Geographic Guide to Birding in North America, hosted by James Currie
- Think Like a Bird: Understanding Bird Behavior, Cornell Lab of Ornithology
- Warbler Identification, Cornell Lab of Ornithology
- Watching Sparrows, Michael Male and Judy Fieth (www.birdfilms.com)

- Watching Warblers, Michael Male and Judy Fieth (www.birdfilms. com)

Apps

- iBirdPro: https://apps.apple.com/ca/app/ibird-pro-guide-to-birds/ id308018823
- Larkwire: https://www.larkwire.com/
- Merlin: https://merlin.allaboutbirds.org/

Articles on Apps (See Notes or References for links)

- *Merlin Bird ID* – Robert Perkins
- *The best birding apps are ones tied to bird guidebooks* – Jim Williams

GEAR

- Binoculars - Nikon Monarch M511 8 x 42
- Field notebook - Rite in the Rain
- Nikon Cool Pix P1000
- Nikon Cool Pix P900

PHYSICAL LOCATIONS
Southern Ontario "fallout" points

- Edgelake in Stoney Creek
- Long Point
- Point Pelee Provincial Park
- Rondeau Provincial Park
- Sedgewick Forest in Oakville

CATS and BIRDS

- A synthesis of human-related avian mortality in Canada: http://dx.doi.org/10.5751/ACE-00581-080211
- Cats and Birds: http://catsandbirds.ca/
- High-cat diet: urban coyotes feast on pets, study finds: https://www.theguardian.com/environment/2019/apr/12/protect-your-pets-cats-make-up-one-fifth-of-coyotes-diet-in-los-angeles

BIRD SPECIALITY STORE

- Wild Birds Unlimited - locally, in Burlington and Guelph, Ontario

22. APPENDIX C: BOOKS ON MINERAL EXPLORATION AND DEVELOPMENT

I realize that mineral exploration and development doesn't really have much to do with this book, but as my pre-Lyme life was devoted to it, it is very interesting to me. Therefore, I want to make these recommendations anyway, for anyone curious to learn more about these topics. Books written on mineral discoveries can make for fascinating reading; they are real-life adventure stories featuring heroes who are driven to succeed, and are often truly eccentric characters. Four in particular stand out for me.

Barren Lands, An Epic Search for Diamonds in the North American Arctic, by Kevin Krajick (2001) is the story of the first discovery of diamond mines in Canada by Chuck Fipke and Stew Blusson. Fragments of kimberlites, the rocks that host diamonds, had been eroded, smeared out and moved by multiple glacial pulses during the last ice age. Not all kimberlites contain diamonds. These intrepid explorers devised proprietary techniques to identify which kimberlite fragments were prospective, that is, derived from potentially diamondiferous kimberlites. They traced the unique geochemical signatures of the diamond host rocks by interpreting and following the correct glacial path back to the bedrock source. In doing so, they battled not only the harsh terrain and climate, but also the competition, beating the world's most famous diamond company, DeBeers, to the punch. In my opinion, they proved that DeBeers was a much better marketer ("a man should spend three months' salary on a diamond ring") than they were explorers.

The second book is called *The Conquest of Copper Mountain*, by Forbes Wilson (1981). It truly is an adventure story, recording one of the world's greatest engineering feats: the discovery and subsequent construction of the Grasberg copper mine in Irian Jaya, Indonesia (now West Papua). This is a story of heroics, leading from the malaria-ridden mangrove swamps at the coastline into the central mountainous spine, 12,000 feet above sea level.

My third recommendation is *The Big Score: Robert Friedland, Inco, and the Voisey's Bay Hustle*, by Jacquie McNish (1998). It is a history of the discovery of the Voisey's Bay copper-nickel deposit in Labrador and subsequent machinations by Robert Friedland as he played Inco off against Falconbridge in a bidding war. I'm not recommending this one just because I'm mentioned in it! I lived through this dramatic, exciting period and know most of the key players. Many are former Inco colleagues I worked with. On behalf of Inco, I had optioned a gold exploration property in Newfoundland from Albert Chislett, the prospector who made the discovery, long before he became one of the richest men in Newfoundland. I'm proud to say that I have a piece of drill core from the discovery hole in my rock collection.

Finally, an almost surreal history called *The Sheltering Desert*, by Henno Martin (1983). This is the tale of two young German geologists who were conducting geological mapping in the wilds of Namibia when the Second World War broke out. Afraid that if they returned to civilization they would be interned, they camped out in the wilderness for two and half years and even continued to conduct geological surveys!

RELATED TITLES

AN IDENTIFICATION GUIDE

This book is a richly detailed photographic guide to the Ducks, Geese, and Swans of North America, including the Hawaiian Islands, Greenland, Mexico and the U.S. Territories in the Pacific Ocean. The photographs, mostly by the author, were selected to highlight plumage phases, age classes and variation and behavioral postures. Brief text describes the different categories of waterfowl and brief bullet points highlight important identification features.

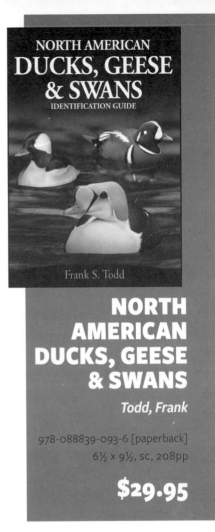

NORTH AMERICAN DUCKS, GEESE & SWANS

Todd, Frank

978-088839-093-6 [paperback]
6½ x 9½, sc, 208pp

$29.95

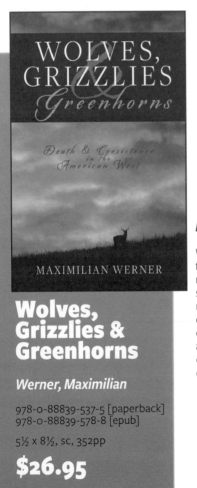

Death & Coexistence in the American West

Werner recounts the two-and-a-half years he spent tracking down and looking after a wolf pack that was rumored to have settled in the Centennial Valley of southwest Montana. Along the way he encounters and reflects on the lives of other animals, including deer, elk, fox, coyote, skunks, and grizzly bears. But he also encounters other humans too—ranchers, hunters, land and wildlife managers, cowboys—who offer their own, often conflicting perspectives about the natural world, other animals, and how both ought to be treated.

Wolves, Grizzlies & Greenhorns

Werner, Maximilian

978-0-88839-537-5 [paperback]
978-0-88839-578-8 [epub]

5½ x 8½, sc, 352pp

$26.95

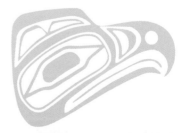

Saving Billions of Birds from Windows

Birds behave as if sheet glass is invisible to them. They kill themselves striking clear and reflective panes in all types and sizes of human-built structures the world over. The killing is indiscriminate, taking the fit and unfit species, of any age category- both common and of conservation concern.

Window-kills occur in the billions worldwide annually. The victims are always unintended, unnecessary, harmless, and have no voice or other means to protect themselves. Unlike the complexities of other environmental challenges, such as climate change, this important conservation issue for birds and people can be solved, and the means to do so are described within the pages of this work to guide this worthy effort.

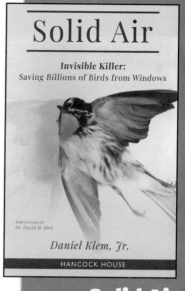

Solid Air

Klem Jr, Daniel

978-0-88839-646-4 [paperback]

978-0-88839-640-2 [hardcover]

978-0-88839-665-5 [epub]

6 x 9, sc, 224pp

$24.95

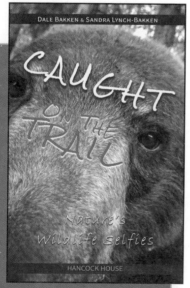

Caught on the Trail

Bakken, Dale & Sandra-Lynch

978-0-88839-058-5 [paperback]

978-0-88839-263-3 [epub]

6 x 9, sc, 160ppc

$24.95

Nature's Wildlife Selfies

Have you ever wondered what roams your backyard in the dead of night? Shares the same nature trail with you, or is living on the fringe of your rural property?

We have. So, we trekked our property, at the base of a mountain in northern British Columbia, and set up game cameras to get our answer! Over a span of seven years, we captured rare photos of wolverines as they fed on a frozen carcass, a sow grizzly and her cub patrolling the trails, coyotes, wolves, and black bears in all colours and sizes as they frolicked, fought and raised young throughout the year.

This book will help the reader gain a better appreciation for the trials and tribulations of wild animals and how to use game cameras and respect the wildlife we seek to capture on camera.

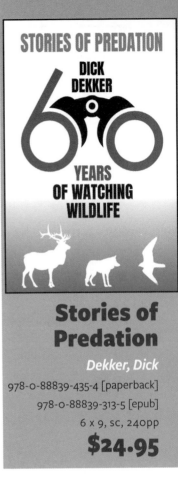
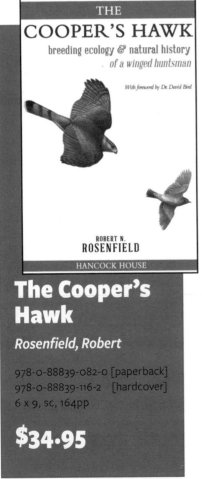